Introducing
Palliative Care

D0494233

Robert Twycross MA, DM, FRCP

Macmillan Clinical Reader in Palliative Medicine,
University of Oxford
Consultant Physician, Sir Michael Sobell House,
Churchill Hospital, Oxford
Senior Research Fellow, St Peter's College, Oxford
Director, WHO Collaborating Centre for Palliative
Cancer Care, Oxford
Chairman, International School for Cancer Care

RADCLIFFE MEDICAL PRESS
OXFORD AND NEW YORK

©1995 Robert Twycross

Radcliffe Medical Press Ltd
18 Marcham Road, Abingdon, Oxon, OX14 1AA, UK

Radcliffe Medical Press, Inc.
141 Fifth Avenue, New York, NY 10010, USA

British Library Cataloguing in Publication Data

A catalogue record for this book is available from the British Library.

ISBN 1 85775 039 X

Library of Congress Cataloging-in-Publication Data

Twycross, Robert G.
    Introducing palliative care / Robert Twycross.
        p.   cm.
    Includes bibliographical references and index.
    ISBN 1-85775-039-X : $22.50
    1. Palliative treatment.   1. Title.
    [DNLM: 1. Palliative Treatment.   2. Terminal Care.   3. Neoplasms–therapy.   4. Neoplasms–psychology.   5. Pain, Intractable–drug therapy.   WB   310 T975i 1995]
    R726.8.T97 1995
    362. 1'75–dc20
    DNLM/DLC
    for Library of Congress   95-3744
                                                                                   CIP

Typeset by AMA Graphics Limited, Preston
Printed and bound in Great Britain by Biddles Ltd, Guildford and King's Lynn

Contents

Preface

This book represents a further stage in the evolution of a set of lecture notes originally prepared over a decade ago for clinical students of the Oxford University Medical School attending a five day course at Sir Michael Sobell House on 'Care of the Patient with Advanced Cancer'. A number of other centres both in the UK and in other countries have also made use of them, in some cases translating them into the local language. Because of the continued interest in the lecture notes, they have been revised and are being published professionally in a format which is easier to handle and which will facilitate their use as a course manual.

Specialist palliative care services are often focused on the care of patients with endstage cancer. The same is true of this book. The general principles and most of the details, however, are applicable to patients dying from other progressive incurable disorders. The content is inevitably selective, notably in relation to symptom management. The book also reflects an emphasis on 'whole person' care, ethics, communication skills, coping with loss, as well as providing an introduction to pain and symptom management.

When compiling a book of this nature, it is necessary to acknowledge many people and sources, some long forgotten. One is reminded of the old saying that, *'There is nothing new under the sun'*. To the anonymous teachers from the past, I express my gratitude. In the pages devoted to communication and breaking bad news, the perceptive reader may well see the more obvious shadows of Ivan Lichter, Susan Le Poidevin, Robert Buckman and Peter Maguire. David Frampton made many useful suggestions, as did Gilly Burn, Karen Jenns, Andrew Wilcock and Angela Williams.

The help of course tutors, past and present, is also acknowledged. These include Jennifer Barraclough, John Barton, Ruben Bild, David

Cook, Ann Couldrick, Ginny Dunn, Michael Minton, Sue Palmer, Marilyn Relf, Victoria Slater, Rosalyn Staveley, and Averil Stedeford. Where a sole or prime author is still clearly identifiable, this is acknowledged in the text.

Robert Twycross
January 1995

Drug names

Generic drug names are generally the same regardless of the country of use. Important exceptions are:

UK	USA
Activated dimethicone	Simethicone
Adrenaline	Epinephrine
Dextropropoxyphene	Propoxyphene
Diamorphine (di-acetylmorphine)	Heroin
Frusemide	Furosemide
Glycopyrronium	Glycopyrrolate
Hyoscine	Scopolamine
Lignocaine	Lidocaine
Liquid paraffin	Mineral oil
Methotrimeprazine	Levomepromazine
Paracetamol	Acetaminophen
Pethidine	Meperidine

In addition readers should note that prednisolone and its inactive prodrug, prednisone, are identical in potency and efficacy.

All the drugs referred to are not universally available. The reader is advised to check with his own National Formulary or drug compendium if he is in doubt.

Diamorphine is available only in the UK and Canada.

List of abbreviations

General

BNF	British National Formulary
BP	British Pharmacopoeia
IASP	International Association for the Study of Pain
UK	United Kingdom
USA	United States of America
WHO	World Health Organization

Medical

CNS	central nervous system
COPD	chronic obstructive pulmonary disease
CSF	cerebrospinal fluid
CT	computed tomography
H_1, H_2	histamine type 1, type 2 receptors
MAOI(s)	mono-amine oxidase inhibitor(s)
MRI	magnetic resonance imaging
NSAID(s)	nonsteroidal anti-inflammatory drug(s)

PCA	patient controlled analgesia
PG(s)	prostaglandin(s)
5HT	5-hydroxytryptamine (serotonin)

Drug administration

b.d.	twice daily; alternative, b.i.d.
daily	once a day
IM	intramuscular
IV	intravenous
m/r	modified release; alternative, slow release
nocte	at bedtime
o.d.	once daily (usually in the morning)
p.c.	post cebus, after meals
PO	per os, by mouth
PR	per rectum, by rectum
q4h, q6h	every 4 hours, every 6 hours etc.
q.d.s.	four times a day; alternative, q.i.d.
SC	subcutaneous
SL	sublingual
stat	immediately
t.d.s.	three times a day; alternative, t.i.d.

Units

cm	centimetre(s)
g	gram(s)
h	hour(s)
Hg	mercury
IU	international unit(s)
kg	kilogram(s)
l	litre(s)
mcg	microgram(s)
mEq	milli-equivalent(s)
mg	milligram(s)
ml	millilitre(s)
mm	millimetre(s)
mmol	millimole(s)
min	minute(s)

PART ONE

General Topics

Fatal statistics · Palliative care
A typical palliative care service
Dying at home
Ethics of palliative care · Hope

Fatal statistics

Cancer is common.

One third of the population in the UK develops cancer.

One quarter of the population in the UK dies of cancer.

These figures are true for all developed countries. The incidence has increased considerably over the last 30 years. It is still increasing because of

- tobacco smoking
- an ageing population.

Despite these gloomy figures, it is important to have a balanced view of cancer because

- some cancers can be cured, possibly as many as one third
- even if incurable, people may survive for many years.

For example, 16% of a group of patients with colorectal cancer noted to have a solitary hepatic metastasis at the time of the initial laparotomy survived 5 years.[1]

Further, it has been shown in breast cancer patients that[2]

- a fighting spirit or denial results in a better prognosis
- fatalism or helplessness/hopelessness results in a worse prognosis.

Palliative care

'Palliative' is derived from a Latin word 'pallium', meaning a cloak or cover. Thus, in palliative care, symptoms are 'cloaked' with treatments whose primary or sole aim is to promote patient comfort.

Definition and scope

Palliative care is the active total care of patients and their families by a multiprofessional team at a time when the patient's disease is no longer responsive to curative treatment and life expectancy is relatively short (Figure 1.1). It responds to physical, psychological, social and spiritual needs, and extends if necessary to support in bereavement (Figure 1.2). The goal of palliative care is to provide support and

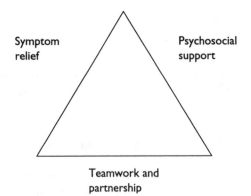

Figure 1.1:   Three essential components of palliative care.

care for patients in the last phases of the disease so that they can live as fully and comfortably as possible.

Although sometimes described as 'low tech and high touch', palliative care is not intrinsically against medical technology. Rather it seeks to ensure that compassion and not science is the controlling force in patient care. 'High tech' investigations and treatments are used only when their benefits clearly outweigh any potential burdens.

Palliative care includes rehabilitation. It seeks to help patients achieve and maintain their maximum potential physically, psychologically, socially and spiritually, however limited these have become as a result of disease progression. Palliative care

- affirms life and regards dying as a normal process
- neither hastens nor postpones death
- provides relief for patients from pain and other distressing symptoms
- integrates psychological, social and spiritual aspects of care so that patients may come to terms with their own death as fully and constructively as they can
- offers a support system to help patients live as actively and creatively as possible until death

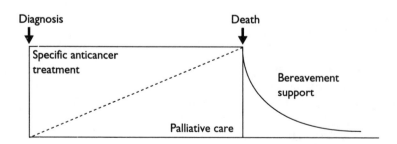

Figure 1.2: Diagram to show the relationship between anticancer treatment and palliative care over time.

- offers a support system to help families cope during the patient's illness and in bereavement
- is often called 'hospice care', particularly in the UK.

Teamwork

Palliative care is best administered by a group of people working as a team. The team is collectively concerned with the total wellbeing of the patient and family. In practice, some or all of the following will be involved

- doctor(s) and nurses (essential 'core' clinical team)
- physiotherapist, occupational therapist, and other specific therapists
- social worker, chaplain/priest/rabbi and/or other advisers
- volunteers.

Because there is an overlap of roles, co-ordination is an important part of teamwork. Conflict inevitably erupts from time to time in a team of highly motivated, skilled professionals. One of the challenges of teamwork is how to handle conflict constructively and creatively.

Partnership

The essence of palliative care is *partnership* between the caring team and the patient and family. Partnership requires mutual respect. Partnership and respect are manifested by

- courtesy in behaviour
- politeness in speech
- not 'patronizing'

- being honest
- listening
- explaining
- agreeing priorities and goals
- discussing treatment options
- accepting treatment refusal.

Taken collectively, the above list provides the basis for an individual approach to care.

> 'Care begins when difference is recognized. I reserve the name "caregivers" for the people who are willing to listen to ill persons and to respond to their individual experiences. Caring has nothing to do with categories. When the caregiver communicates to the ill person that she cares about the patient's uniqueness, she makes the person's life meaningful.'[3]

Quality of life

'Quality of life is what a person says it is.'

It is often said that the goal of palliative care is the highest possible quality of life for both patient and family. Quality of life refers to subjective satisfaction experienced and/or expressed by an individual; it relates to and is influenced by all the dimensions of personhood – physical, psychological, social and spiritual.

There is good quality of life when the aspirations of an individual are matched and fulfilled by present experience. There is poor quality of life when there is a wide divergence between aspirations and present experience.[4] To improve quality of life, it is necessary to narrow the gap between aspirations and what is possible (Figure 1.3).

Thus, a tetraplegic ex-gymnastics instructor is able to say, 'The quality of my life is excellent, though to see me you wouldn't believe it. I've come to terms with my loss and discovered the powers of my mind.' And a 30 year-old man dying of disseminated osteosarcoma complicated by paraplegia comments, 'The last year of my life has been the best.'

Quality of life scores tend to be flawed because they measure only selected aspects and not global subjective satisfaction.[5–7]

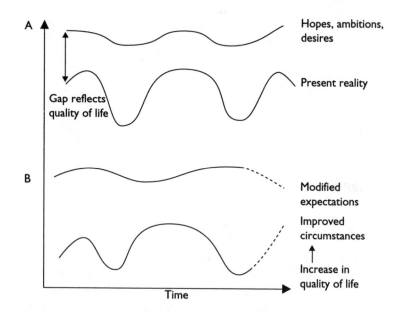

Figure 1.3: A: a representation of the gap between reality and hopes. B: improvement in quality of life represents either a reduction in expectations or a change in present reality.[4]

A typical palliative care service

Although focusing on home care, most palliative care services in the UK offer a range of services

- specialist home care nurses
- medical consultations:
    at home with the general practitioner
    in other wards and hospitals
- outpatient clinics
- day care
- inpatient care
- bereavement support
- education (usually)
- research (sometimes).

Clinical services are directed by a medical director/consultant physician and a matron/senior nurse. Typically, about 95% of patients have cancer. Although there is a provider contract with one or more health authority, a variable amount of money needs to be raised annually to make ends meet – anything from 30 to 70% of the total cost of the service.

Home care

Specialist home care nurses (Macmillan nurses) liaise with the primary health care team and offer advice on treatment and care. Because they provide support for the whole family, more patients are able to remain at home until death.

Day care

A day centre receives 10 to 15 patients a day. Patients are driven to and from the centre by volunteers. Patients att :nd for social support and to give the family a break. Medical and nursing care is also available. Services include bathing, hairdressing, manicure, chiropody and massage. The day centre enables many patients to remain at home for much longer than would otherwise be possible.

Patients attending a day centre often find new meaning and purpose in living as they make new friends, explore opportunities for creative expression, and enjoy cultural activities together.

Inpatient care

Patients are admitted for symptom management, for family relief (respite) or to die. About half of all admissions end with the patient returning home or to relatives. A high nurse–patient ratio is maintained because the physical and psychological needs of the patients are often considerable.

Rehabilitation is facilitated by an occupational therapist and a physiotherapist. Inpatients are encouraged to make use of the facilities of the day centre. The median length of stay is typically eight to ten days.

Bereavement support

This may be provided by trained volunteers under the supervision of a social worker. They offer support to a number of bereaved relatives and other key carers. Support may also be continued after bereavement by the home care nurses.

Voluntary help

The support provided by a specialist palliative care service is enhanced by volunteers who are involved in many aspects of the care. Volunteers receive initial and continuing inservice training.

Education and research

Education is an important aspect of palliative care. Various courses give opportunities for other health care professionals to learn how to care better for dying patients.

Research is important if the care of dying patients is to be improved further. It is time-consuming and costly, and is undertaken by only a small number of units.

Dying at home

Most people, if given the opportunity, would choose to die at home rather than in the alien environment of a hospital. With good support services, high quality care is often possible at home and may well be more appropriate for the patient and family.

Prerequisites for good home care

Any or all of the following may be required

- primary health care team:
  general practitioner
  community nurse
- community care services

- specialist support team:
  home care nurse
  palliative care physician
  social worker
  clinical psychologist/psychotherapist
  occupational therapist

- priest/rabbi, etc.

- friends or volunteers to sit with the patient while the key carer goes shopping or has 'time off'

- day care

- outpatient evaluation

- night nurses

- short periods of inpatient care:
  for symptom management
  to give the family a rest (respite).

Ethics of palliative care

The ethics of palliative care are those of medicine in general. Doctors have a dual responsibility, namely to preserve life and to relieve suffering. At the end of life, relief of suffering is of even greater importance as preserving life becomes increasingly impossible.

Four cardinal principles[8]

- patient autonomy (respect for the patient as a person)

- beneficence (do good)

- nonmaleficence (minimize harm)

- justice (fair use of available resources).

The four cardinal principles need to be applied against a background of

- respect for life
- acceptance of the ultimate inevitability of death.

In practice, these comprise three dichotomies which need to be applied in a balanced manner. Thus

- the potential benefits of treatment must be balanced against the potential burdens
- striving to preserve life but, when biologically futile, providing comfort in dying
- individual needs are balanced against those of society.

Appropriate treatment

All patients must die eventually. Part of the art of medicine is to decide when sustaining life is essentially futile and, therefore, when to allow death to occur without further impediment. Thus, in palliative care, the primary aim of treatment is not to prolong life but to make the life which remains as comfortable and as meaningful as possible.

A doctor is not obliged legally or ethically to preserve life 'at all costs'. Rather, life should be sustained when from a biological point of view it is sustainable. Priorities change when a patient is clearly dying. There is no obligation to employ treatments if their use can best be described as prolonging the process of dying. A doctor has neither a duty nor the right to prescribe a lingering death.

It is not a question of to treat or not to treat but what is the most appropriate treatment given the patient's biological prospects and his personal and social circumstances. Appropriate treatment for an acutely ill patient may be inappropriate in the dying (Figures 1.4 and 1.5).

Nasogastric tubes, IV infusions, antibiotics, cardiac resuscitation, and artificial respiration are all primarily support measures for use in acute or acute-on-chronic illnesses to assist a patient through the initial crisis towards recovery of health. To use such measures in patients who are close to death and in whom there is no expectation of a return to health is usually inappropriate (and therefore bad medicine).

Medical care is a continuum, ranging from complete cure at one end to symptom relief at the other. Many types of treatment span the entire spectrum, notably radiotherapy and, to a lesser extent, chemotherapy and surgery. It is important to keep the therapeutic aim clearly in mind with any form of treatment. In deciding what is appropriate, the key points are

- the patient's biological prospects
- the therapeutic aim and benefits of each treatment

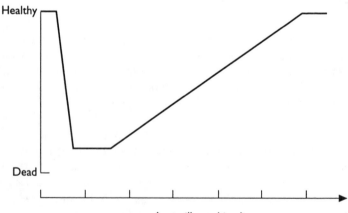

Figure 1.4: A graphical representation of acute illness. Biological prospects are generally good. Acute resuscitative measures are important and enable the patient to survive the initial crisis. Recovery is aided by the natural forces of healing; rehabilitation is completed by the patient on his own, without continued medical support.

- the adverse effects of treatment
- the need not to prescribe a lingering death.

Although the possibility of unexpected improvement or recovery should not be ignored, there are many occasions when it is appropriate to 'give death a chance'.

As a person becomes terminally ill, or severely limited physically and mentally as a result of senile decay, his interest in hydration and nutrition often becomes minimal. Because the natural outcome of both incurable progressive disease and advanced senility is death, these are circumstances in which it is wrong to force a patient to accept food and fluid. The patient's disinterest or positive disinclination should be seen as part of the process of 'letting go'.

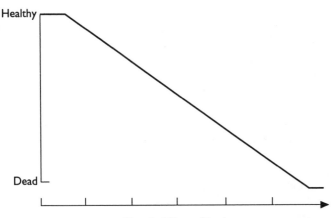

Figure 1.5:   A graphical representation of terminal illness. Biological prospects progressively worsen. Acute and terminal illnesses are therefore distinct pathophysiological entities. Therapeutic interventions that can best be described as prolonging the distress of dying are futile and inappropriate.

Hope

'Hope is an expectation greater than zero of achieving a goal.'

Hope needs an object. Setting realistic goals jointly with a patient is one way of restoring and maintaining hope. This can be initiated by asking the patient, 'And what do you hope will come out of this consultation?'.

It may be necessary to break down an ultimate (probably unrealistic) goal into a series of (more realistic) mini-goals. Thus, if a patient says, 'I want to be cured' or a paraplegic says, 'I want to walk again', an initial reply could be:

> 'I hear what you are saying . . . but that, I suppose, is your ultimate goal. I think it might be helpful if we could agree on a series of more short term goals. Reaching these would give us all a sense of achievement. Does that seem sensible to you?'

Setting goals is an integral part of caring for patients with an incurable disease, including terminal cancer. In one study, doctors and nurses in palliative care units set significantly more goals than did their counterparts in a general hospital.[9]

Hope is also related to other aspects of life and relationships (Table 1.1). Communication of painful truth does not equal destruction of hope (*see* p.22). Hope of recovery is replaced by an alternative hope.

In patients close to death, hope tends to become focused on

- being rather than achieving
- relationship with others
- relationship with God or a 'higher being'.

Table 1.1:   Factors that influence hope in the terminally ill

Decrease	Increase
Feeling devalued	Feeling valued
Abandonment and isolation 'conspiracy of silence' 'there is nothing more which can be done'	Meaningful relationship(s) reminiscence humour
Lack of direction/goals	Realistic goals
Unrelieved pain and discomfort	Pain and symptom relief

It is possible for hope to increase when a person is close to death, provided care and comfort remain satisfactory.[10] When there is little else left to hope for, it is still realistic to hope

- not to be left alone to die
- for a peaceful death.

Psychosocial Aspects of Care

Communication

'Communications, like tumours, may be benign or malignant. They may also be invasive, and the effects of bad communication with a patient may metastasize to the family. Truth is one of the most powerful therapeutic agents available to us, but we still need to develop a proper understanding of its clinical pharmacology and to recognize optimum timing and dosage in its use. Similarly, we need to understand the closely related metabolisms of hope and denial.'[11]

The aims of communication are to

- reduce uncertainty
- enhance relationships
- give the patient and family a direction in which to move.

The basic message a patient wants to hear at a time of increasing uncertainty is:

'No matter what happens to you, we will not desert you.' (acceptance)

'You may be dying, but you are still important to us.' (affirmation)

Only part of this can be said in words:

'We can relieve your pain and can ease most other symptoms.'

'I will see you regularly.'

'One of us will always be available.'

'Let's work out how best we can help you and your family.'

A large part of the message is conveyed to the patient by nonverbal means. Nonverbal communication includes

- facial expression
- eye contact
- posture, including whether sitting or standing
- pitch and pace of voice
- touch.

Touch is an important means of conveying re-assurance and comfort, e.g. holding a patient's hand – although cultural norms must be borne in mind.

Getting started

- make time for an unhurried conversation without interruption
- privacy is important
- introduce self by name and shake hands
- sit down to indicate you have time to listen
- make eye contact
- avoid medical jargon.

A patient-led agenda is particularly important in patients with many symptoms. A formal systematic enquiry alone may leave the doctor uncertain as to what to tackle first – and add to the patient's distress by failing to develop a clear plan of campaign. Useful ways of starting include:

'What do you hope will come out of this consultation?'

'Can you tell me about your problems?'

'How are your feeling?'

It is often helpful to allow a new patient to tell her story from the time the illness first manifested – even if this was several years ago, e.g. 'We have not met before. It would help me if you could start right from the beginning'. This often throws up unresolved concerns or resentments from the past which may be crucial to present management and support.

Active listening

- nod from time to time to show that you are still paying attention
- if the patient stops in the middle of a sentence, repeat her last three words; this gives permission to continue, and the offer is usually accepted

- pick up on cues, e.g. 'It's like Granny's illness', 'What do you mean – "It's like Granny's illness"?'

- keep the interview focused

- reflect questions back, e.g. 'What do *you* think the operation was for?'

- ask about feelings, e.g. 'How did/does that make you feel?'

- validate feelings, e.g. 'It's natural you should feel like that'

- watch body language and pick up on nonverbal cues

- summarize and check the accuracy of your understanding of the patient's problems

- if there is a long list of problems, ask the patient to prioritize them.

Asking questions

One of the primary aims of a consultation is to elicit the patient's feelings and concerns. Some questions tend to restrict the amount of information shared by the patient. Thus

- *leading questions* tend to produce the answer the questioner wants to hear, e.g. 'Are you feeling better today?'

- *closed questions* tend to produce the answer yes or no, e.g. 'Have you any pain?'

- *open questions* allow the patient to express feelings and concerns, e.g. 'How are you feeling?' and 'Can you tell me what's been happening since we last met?'.

Without open questions, it is usually impossible to discover how the patient is really feeling, and find out what the main concerns are.

Avoid distancing

Distancing is behaviour by which caregivers avoid becoming involved with a patient on a psychosocial level, usually without being aware of it. Common ways by which doctors distance themselves include

- nonverbal messages:
  always busy
  general demeanour
  facial expression
  tone of voice

- placing people in diagnostic categories, e.g. 'She's a breast cancer' or 'He's a difficult patient'

- never enquiring beyond the physical, i.e. never asking, 'How are you coping?' or 'How are you feeling?'

- closed questions

- deflecting patient's questions

- paying selective attention to 'safe' physical aspects:
  Patient 'I am worried about myself. I am losing weight and the pain in my back has come back again'
  Doctor 'Tell me about the pain'

- premature normalization, e.g. by saying when a patient starts to cry, 'Don't worry, everyone in your position feels upset' instead of, 'I can see you're upset. Can you bear to tell me exactly what is upsetting you?'

- premature or false re-assurance, e.g. 'Don't worry. You leave it to me. Everything will be all right'

- using euphemisms to mislead

- 'jollying along'/expecting the patient to keep up a brave face, e.g. 'Come on, the sun's shining; there's no need to look so glum!'.

Breaking bad news

Bad news is information that drastically and unpleasantly alters a patient's view of her future. In practice, it is seldom a question of 'to tell or not to tell', but more a matter of 'when and how to tell'.

Breaking bad news usually causes distress to both the patient and the newsgiver. It is necessary to be prepared for a strong emotional reaction, e.g. tears, anger. Telling the patient and family together avoids difficulties and mistrust. It also gives opportunity for mutual support.

The principle 'never destroy hope' is sometimes used as a reason for not informing a patient of the seriousness of the situation. False optimism is a potent destroyer of hope. On the other hand, a total catharsis by the doctor of all that is negative either to the patient or to the family may irreversibly destroy hope and result in intractable anxiety and despair. It is necessary to apply two parallel principles, namely

- never lie to a patient
- avoid thoughtless candour.

Gradual communication of the truth within the context of continued support and encouragement almost always leads to enhancement of hope (*see* p.14).

> *The doctor-patient relationship is founded on trust.*
> *It is fostered by honesty but poisoned by deceit.*

The doctor's relationship with the patient should not be compromised by making unwise (and unethical) promises to the relatives about not informing the patient. It is necessary to check awareness, i.e. determine where the patient is at present in terms of knowledge and understanding, and to proceed according to her responses.

If a patient indicates directly or indirectly that she does not wish to regard her illness as fatal, it is wrong to force the truth on her. She is using denial as a coping strategy and, as such, it is vital to present wellbeing. Few patients adopt such a stance permanently.

Patients who want to know more about their condition often ask indirectly:

'And what's the next step, doctor?'

'How long do you reckon this will go on, doctor?'

'I'm not getting any better, am I?'

Sometimes a doctor needs to use open questions to find out if a patient wants more information:

'What things have been running through your mind as to the cause of your symptoms?'

'This illness is dragging on. Are there times when you find yourself looking on the black side?'

Alternatively, it may be helpful to ask the patient:

'Are you the sort of person who likes to know what's happening or do you like to leave it all to the doctor?'

If the patient indicates they prefer to 'leave it to the doctors', this should be accepted as the *present* position. Permission should be given, however, to ask questions at any time should the patient wish to.

If the patient wants more information

- give a 'warning shot' before stating the diagnosis, e.g. 'Tests indicate that we could be dealing with something serious'
- tailor the information to the patient's perceived needs
- use a hierarchy of euphemisms:
  'some abnormal cells'

    'a kind of tumour'
    'a bit cancerous'

- be prepared to stop if the patient indicates that she has heard enough, e.g. 'Well, I'll leave all that in your hands, doctor'

- explore how she *feels* about the situation.

    Doctors generally underestimate what a patient already knows.

For most people, cancer is an emotive word. If asked directly 'Have I got cancer?', first discover what the patient understands by 'cancer'. If to the patient it means an agonizing death, it is important before confirming the diagnosis to explain that this need not be because treatments are now available to relieve pain and other symptoms should they develop.

After giving bad news, try to offer some good news – but not before finding out how the patient feels about the bad news. Good news might include

- what can be done to relieve pain and other symptoms

- there will still be good times despite the progressive illness.

Truth has a broad spectrum with gentleness at one end and harshness at the other. Patients prefer gentle truth. As far as possible, soften the initial impact of emotionally negative words:

    Not 'You've got cancer.'   *But* 'Tests indicate that it is a form of cancer.'

    Not 'You've got three months to live.'   *But* 'Time is probably limited.'

Use words with positive rather than negative overtones:

    Not 'You've got weaker.'   *But* 'Energy, at the moment, is limited.'

Not 'Things are getting worse.' *But* 'Things don't seem to be so good this week.'

Euphemisms are legitimate if used to express truth gently; they are wrong if used to deceive.

Dealing with anger

Anger is a normal response to bad news and may be directed at the doctor. It is important not to become defensive. Instead, listen carefully to what is being expressed, clarify the causes and indicate that, 'Given what has been happening to you, I'm not surprised you feel so angry'. Judgements about the appropriateness of the focus of the anger are not helpful.

In summary

- get the physical surroundings right, e.g. privacy
- establish what the patient knows and what she wants to know
- use open questions
- the initial blow may be softened by stressing what medical science can offer, perhaps erring on the side of optimism
- do not give false hope
- do not be afraid of silence
- pay attention to reactions
- check back to ensure that the message has been taken in
- make sure you are answering the question being asked
- try to get the patient to come to her own conclusion

- do not give more information than is wanted
- accept denial but do not collude with it, e.g. 'Perhaps we'd better just wait and see'
- have the confidence to say, 'I don't know'
- allow expression of strong emotion, e.g. tears, anger
- acknowledge the awfulness of uncertainty and explore the problems it creates
- establish a positive direction in which to move
- not talking does not prevent the inevitable from happening
- be honest with yourself; when someone says he wants to protect the patient, he is often trying to protect himself.

Strategies for coping with uncertainty

Prognosis depends on many different factors – both physical and psychological. Although mean and median figures for survival are available, these relate to 'Mr Average' and not to the patient in your consultation room. When a patient asks about prognosis, try to avoid giving a specific length of time:

> Patient 'How long have I got, doctor?'
>
> Doctor 'I don't know – and nobody knows . . . there are just too many factors to take into account – both physical and psychological . . . I don't know.'

Many terminally ill patients die sooner than the doctor's estimate.[12] If given a specific time, some patients act as if the doctor's estimate is divine prophecy. In consequence, they become increasingly fearful as the 'deadline' approaches and, indeed, may suffer some non-cancerous catastrophe on the day of their predicted death – and die.

Having established that nobody knows, it is important to

- ask the patient what made him ask. This may unearth specific concerns which can then be discussed
- acknowledge that *living with uncertainty* can be very difficult, e.g. 'That's hard isn't it . . . having to live with the uncertainty'
- discuss coping strategies:
  a rolling horizon
  hope for the best but plan for the worst
  reaching anniversaries
  living one day at a time.

A rolling horizon

Here the anticipated survival is four to six months or more:

> 'Given how you are now, you should work on the basis that you will be well enough to do what you want to do for the next two/three months. So go home and fill your diary out for this period of time – with the high expectation that you will be able to fulfil your commitments. If in four weeks time, you are still as good as you are now or better, then fill your diary out for another month, and so on.'

Hope for the best but plan for the worst

Here the anticipated survival is two to three months, possibly more:

> 'Given how things have been and are now, it is difficult to plan confidently for the future. What I suggest is that you adopt a "cross-eyed" approach. With one eye plan as if things are going to work out fairly well and, with the other, make alternative plans in case things work out not so well . . . How does that seem to you?'

Reaching anniversaries

Here the outlook seems very poor, but the patient is still hoping for some time. In this circumstance, it may help to identify anniversaries or special events which will occur in the next few months, and suggest to the patient that she should aim to reach them one by one.

Living one day at a time

Some people do this successfully for months, but it can lead to wasted time and opportunities because the patient sets no medium term goals. However, in people who are within a few weeks of death, it is often a helpful strategy. An alternative is to suggest living one or two weeks at a time.

Beware the tendency of some patients to 'extremize':

> *Doctor* 'It could be two or three months, or it could be two or three years.'
>
> *Patient* (later to family) 'The doctor said I had only two months to live.' *or* 'The doctor said I had at least five years.'

When pressed for more information, remember

- if deteriorating *month by month*, the prognosis is likely to be *months*
- if deteriorating *week by week*, the prognosis is likely to be *weeks*
- If deteriorating *day by day*, the prognosis is likely to be *days.*

But how long is *months, weeks, days* ?

Psychological aspects of terminal illness

Responses to loss

Similar psychological responses occur in various circumstances, ranging from loss of a job, amputation, divorce or bereavement to the anticipated loss of one's own life. They include

- shock
- emotional numbness
- denial
- anger
- anxiety
- guilt
- grief
- resignation or acceptance.

These responses do not necessarily occur in sequence. Several may occur together and some may not occur at all. In cancer patients, more marked responses may be seen

- when the diagnosis is first made
- at the time of the first recurrence
- at each major sign of disease progression.

There is no one right way of responding and adjusting to a poor prognosis. The doctor's task is to help the patient adjust in the best way possible, given that particular patient's background – familial, cultural and spiritual. Many people have a combination of inner resources and good support from the family and others which enable them to cope without prolonged and disabling distress.

Psychological problems

About 50% of palliative care patients experience significant psychological problems. Problems are also common among patients' relatives.

Denial

Denial is a common defence mechanism in the dying. It signifies an ability to obliterate or minimize threatening reality by ignoring it. It may be associated with physiological and other nonverbal evidence of anxiety. With time, most patients make less use of denial, although they may never totally discard it. Patients experience conflict between the wish to know the truth, so that they can prepare themselves and take appropriate action, and the wish to avoid anxiety. Denial is one way they may resolve this. Intervention may be needed when denial persists and interferes with

- the acceptance of treatment
- planning for the future
- relationships.

Anger

Anger may be an appropriate short term reaction to the diagnosis of serious illness, but persistent anger is a problem. If displaced on to the family or staff, it tends to alienate those who want to care. Anger can also interfere with the acceptance of limitations, and may stop a patient from making positive adjustments to physical disability.

Anxiety

Anxiety often relates to uncertainty and fear of the future, and the threat of separation from loved ones. It may present with physical symptoms such as nausea or diarrhoea, rather than with psychological complaints. Many anxious patients sleep badly, have frightening dreams or are reluctant to be left alone at night. Explanation about the illness and special techniques such as relaxation training are the most helpful forms of management but some patients also need anxiolytic drugs. If depressive symptoms are present as well, a sedative anti-depressant drug should be used.

Depression

Recognizing clinically depressed patients is important because they often have a good response to antidepressant drugs. Depression is often missed because symptoms overlap with appropriate grief about dying (sadness) and with the somatic symptoms of cancer, i.e. anorexia, constipation, weight loss. Many patients also try to hide their negative feelings. Pointers to depression include

- persistent low mood (but diurnal variation)
- loss of interest and inability to feel pleasure
- feelings of guilt or unworthiness
- hopelessness/despair
- physical manifestations of anxiety (sweating, tremor, panic)
- suicide attempts.

Paranoid states

Paranoid states may be caused by corticosteroids, a biochemical disturbance or the psychological mechanism of projection – unable to accept that he is dying, the patient believes there is a plot to kill him or that the treatment is the cause of his deterioration.

Communication between patients, staff and families

Staff may not give as much information as patients and families need, even when asked directly. Within families, there is a conflict between the wish to confide and to receive emotional and practical support, and the wish to protect others from distress, particularly children or frail parents. A conspiracy of silence is a source of tension. It blocks discussion of the future and preparation for parting. If it is not resolved, the bereaved often experience much regret.

Other

Cancer related e.g. difficulty in accepting a colostomy, paraplegia or the effects of cerebral secondaries.
Role adjustment may lead to conflict between family members.

Treatment related e.g. adverse drug effects such as hair loss.
Patients may want to share in decisions about when to stop treatment aimed at prolonging life. Fear of death may make some want to go on even when adverse effects are severe and the chance of improvement is minimal. Others may wish to opt for a shorter life of better quality when doctors are advocating more aggressive measures.

Concurrent e.g. a bereavement, or a pre-existing psychiatric illness.

Management

Some psychological problems could be prevented by

- good staff-patient communication, giving information according to individual need
- good staff-patient relationships, with continuity of care
- enabling patients to have some control over the management of their illness.

Psychological problems are easily overlooked by doctors and nurses. Questions such as 'How are you feeling?' and 'How are you coping?' may facilitate the expression of much negative emotion. Alternatively, suspicions that there is a high level of anxiety or severe depression may be confirmed by asking the patient to complete a standard screening test such as the Hospital Anxiety and Depression (HAD) Scale.

Anxiolytics and/or antidepressants are often necessary adjuncts to psychological and social measures. Appropriate treatment will enable the patient to

- have a better quality of life during the illness
- prepare for death
- retain individuality and self-respect to the end.

Care of the relatives

The care of the family is an integral part of the care of the dying. A contented family increases the likelihood of a contented patient. Relative-doctor communication generally needs to be initiated and maintained by the doctor. It is easy to neglect the family because they are reluctant to trouble the doctor 'because he's so busy'.

Telling the relatives

For the family and patient to be too far out of step in relation to knowledge about the diagnosis and the prognosis can create a barrier between them. A common initial reaction is 'You won't tell him, will you, doctor?' or 'We'd prefer you not to tell him, doctor'. This should be seen as an initial shock reaction, stemming from the relative's own instinctive fear of death coupled with a desire to protect a loved one from hurt. It should not be used as an excuse for saying nothing to the patient.

If the family and patient are to be mutually supportive it is necessary to help the relatives move forward from this initial reaction to a position of greater openness and trust. *The family cannot forbid the doctor from discussing diagnosis and prognosis with the patient.* Indeed, given the ethic of medical confidentiality, it is clear that relatives can be told only with the implicit or explicit permission of the patient, and not the other way round.

In practice, there is much to be said for joint interviews at the time of diagnosis and later – patient, relative, doctor and nurse. This prevents collusion and a conspiracy of silence by which the patient is excluded from the process of information sharing. In addition, the presence of a nurse facilitates subsequent clarification of what the doctor said.

The doctor should also make an opportunity to see both the patient and the close family apart from each other. Further separate or joint interviews can then be arranged as necessary. As with the patient, it is generally not necessary or wise initially to tell the family the whole truth (as you perceive it) at one time. The relatives also need time to adjust to the implications of the diagnosis.

Involvement in inpatient care

Admission to hospital or a palliative care unit may be seen as a defeat by the family. It helps if the doctor emphasizes that he is surprised that they have managed to cope for so long and that now, with the need for constant 'round the clock' care, it is impossible for them to continue without a break. It should be emphasized that the presence of relatives and close friends is regarded as important for the patient's continued wellbeing. If practical, unrestricted visits should be encouraged.

The relatives' separation anxiety may be reduced by encouraging them to help in the care of the patient, e.g. adjusting pillows, refilling a water jug, helping with a blanket bath, assisting at meals if necessary. Some relatives need to be taught how to visit, to behave as they would at home, e.g. sit and read a book or newspaper, knit, watch the television together. It may need to be emphasized that a tiring patter of conversation does not have to be kept up.

Overnight accommodation should be arranged when necessary, possibly using a divan in the patient's room or guest accommodation if available and convenient.

Planning for discharge

A proportion of patients with terminal illness, particularly cancer, improve following admission as a result of pain and symptom management. They become physically independent and no longer need to be inpatients.

Many relatives have fears about what will happen should the patient be discharged. A daytime visit or a weekend at home often does much to allay their fear – or confirms after all that discharge is impractical. A doctor (as well as other team members) should discuss matters with the relatives both before and after a trial period at home. Future plans can then be made on the basis of comments by both the family and the patient.

Patients are sometimes overprotected by their family. For example, even though still capable of driving, visiting the pub or betting shop, they are not allowed to do so. It is necessary in these cases to help the relatives to accept the patient's need (and right) to maintain the maximum possible degree of independence. An explanation that a sudden dramatic deterioration is unlikely will help ease the family's apprehension. They also need clear guidance about what to do in an emergency, i.e. whether to call the general practitioner or the hospital/palliative care unit.

Explanation of treatment

Terminally, it is advisable to tell the relatives that, because the patient is less well and swallowing is difficult, medicine may need to be given by injection to prevent pain (or other distress) recurring. If pneumonia develops, the doctor should explain that he plans to treat it symptomatically and not use antibiotics.

After the patient's death

Because bereavement has both a morbidity and a mortality, palliative care does not end when the patient dies. Many relatives have false feelings of guilt:

'If only I'd done this!'

'Do you think, if he'd gone to the hospital sooner, he wouldn't have died?'

Opportunity should be given for such feelings to be aired and questions raised.

Spiritual care

'Palliative care integrates psychological, social and spiritual aspects of care so that patients may come to terms with their own death as fully and constructively as they can.'

Spiritual relates to values (ultimate issues and life principles) and to a person's search for meaning and purpose in life. It also refers to experiences which transcend sensory phenomena.

Religion is a framework of theistic beliefs and rituals which give expression to spiritual concerns.

The spiritual dimension may also be viewed as the integrating component, holding together the physical, psychological and social dimensions (Figure 2.1).

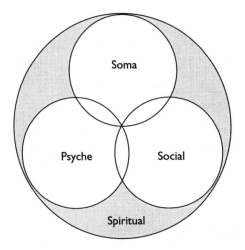

Figure 2.1:   Total care for a person involves four dimensions.

For those nearing the end of life, there is commonly an increased or renewed need for

- affirmation and acceptance
- forgiveness and reconciliation
- the discovery of meaning and direction.

Death is not the ultimate tragedy of life. The ultimate tragedy is depersonalization, e.g.

- dying in an alien and sterile area
- separation from the spiritual nourishment of a fellow human being
- hopelessness and despair.

Glimpses of spirituality at Sobell House[13]

In talking together at Sobell House about spirituality, a rich mixture of experiences, insights and feelings has emerged which defies simple definition. There is both meaning and mystery, a sense of interconnectedness and relationship alongside an awareness of our individuality.

We may connect with the spiritual dimension through the beauty of the natural world, through our relationships with others, through religious practices, through painting or music, or other forms of art. But there is also a sense of awe and aloneness on this journey. We may have faith, and we may search and question. Our feelings may shift from courage and hope to fear – and back again. There may be joy, love, forgiveness and truth, as well as pain and suffering. Through all, a dynamic energy takes us along our different paths. It is an area of experience where we may have more to learn from patients and relatives than we have to teach, more to receive than to give.

Whether apparent or not, most patients are in need of spiritual help and are seeking answers:[14]

Meaning of suffering and pain Why do I have to suffer? Why has this happened to me?

Value systems What value is there in money, material possessions, and social position?

Quest after God Is there a God? Why does God allow me to suffer like this?

The meaning of life What is the meaning of life in a time of serious illness? What's the point of it all?

Guilt feelings I have done many wrong things. How can they be corrected? How can I be forgiven?

Life after death Is there life after death? How can I believe in life after death? What is it like?

Although relatively few patients discuss the spiritual aspects of life and death with their doctor, the majority do so with another team member or with relatives and close friends. It is important to be aware that the dying do consider such issues, and to be able to respond sympathetically if a patient chooses to raise them. Patients are very perceptive and they are unlikely to embarrass a doctor if they sense that communication at this level will cause discomfort.

A doctor's primary responsibility is to help maintain an environment which is supportive of the patient. This includes the relief of symptoms so that the patient is able to reflect on life and its meaning. It is important not to fall into the trap of thinking that you understand the spiritual pain the patient is suffering. Further, it is not generally helpful if a doctor tries to provide neat answers to a patient's questions. Ultimately, each one has to find answers which are personally satisfying. Sharing in not knowing is more comforting than being left feeling other people have all the answers.

When appropriate, the doctor should alert the chaplain/priest/rabbi to the fact that 'Mr Brown is seriously ill and may appreciate a visit'. Respect for the patient as a person does not allow the imposition on him of one's own faith (or lack of it). Many patients are comforted by the discovery that their doctor has a religious faith.

Some possible indicators of spiritual need, pain or dis-ease[15]

- a sense of hopelessness, meaninglessness, powerlessness, e.g. 'I'd be better off dead than living like this'. Such a patient may become withdrawn and suicidal

- intense suffering, e.g. 'I can't endure this any more' and 'What's the point of going on like this?' Includes loneliness, isolation, vulnerability. Challenges the care being given, e.g. 'If this is the best you can do, I'd rather be dead'

- remoteness of God, inability to trust, break with religious and cultural ties, e.g. 'I don't believe in God any more', 'I can't ask him for help' and 'How can I trust people if even God has let me down?'

- anger towards God, religion, clergy, e.g. 'Why? Why me?' and 'What have I done to deserve this?'

- undue stoicism and desire to show others how to do it, e.g. 'I must not let God/my church/my family down'

- a sense of guilt or shame, i.e. illness means punishment; bitter and unforgiving of self/others, e.g. 'I don't deserve to get better'

- concern with moral/ethical nature of treatment. Feelings of unworthiness may relate to guilt and shame, e.g. 'Do you think I should have this treatment/operation? I've had my life'

- unresolved feelings about death manifesting as fear of sleep and the dark, i.e. the longer you stay awake the longer you put off death. Any illness may concentrate the mind and raise questions of what is beyond death, e.g. 'Letting go into what?'

Evaluation

Nonverbal behaviour

- observe affect, e.g. does the person's affect or attitude convey loneliness, depression, anger, agitation or anxiety?

- observe behaviours, e.g. does the person pray and/or does he make use of religious reading material?

Verbal behaviour

- does the person seem to complain out of proportion to his illness?

- are there reports of sleeping difficulties?

- are unusually high doses of sedation or pain medication needed?

- does the person refer to God in any way?

- does the person talk about:
  prayer, faith, hope or anything of a religious nature?
  church functions which are part of his life?

- does the person express concern about the meaning of life?

Environment

- does the person have visitors from church? Are they supportive or do they seem to leave the person feeling upset?

- does the person have with him:
  religious reading material?
  religious medals or other religious objects?

- has the person received religious get well cards?

- does the person use religious pictures, artwork or music to keep his spirits up?

Religious and cultural needs
(John Barton)

'**Respect for privacy, dignity and religious and cultural beliefs.** The [Patient's] Charter Standard is that all health services should make provision so that proper personal consideration is shown to you, for example by ensuring that your privacy, dignity and religious and cultural beliefs are respected.'[16]

For many people, religion is an important element in their lives, from which they derive inspiration and strength.

Every society develops a set of arrangements to enable members to live peacefully with each other. These arrangements form part of that society's culture. Thus, a culture may be defined as the way of living adopted by a specific group of people.

It is important to reach an understanding with each patient and her relatives about religious and cultural needs. People should be cared for where they are in their beliefs and not where we happen to be.

Christianity

Belief in God revealed in Jesus Christ and at work in people and events in the world today through the Holy Spirit. The Church is the worshipping community of believers. God's grace and strength is given in many ways, particularly through the Bible, prayers and sacraments.

Most hospitals have a chapel and many patients value its peace and quiet, e.g. 'I feel a lot better after sitting here in the chapel'.

Three chaplains are appointed in most hospitals:

Church of England (Anglican)
Roman Catholic
Free Church – includes Methodist, Baptist, United Reformed, Congregational, Salvation Army, Moravian, Brethren, Society of Friends (Quakers), Pentecostal, Seventh Day Adventist.

Adherents of certain sects, e.g. Christian Scientists, Jehovah's Witnesses and Mormons, may be reluctant to be seen by a hospital chaplain.

Judaism

Belief in one universal God who is to be worshipped. The Jewish Sabbath is from Friday evening until Saturday evening. There are a number of important Jewish Festivals during the year:

Pesach (first day of Passover – April)
Shavuot (Feast of Weeks – May)
Rosh Hashanah (Jewish New Year – September)
Yom Kippur (Day of Atonement – September)
Succoth (first day of the Feast of Tabernacles – October).

Orthodox Jews eat meat only when it has been killed by their own trained people (Kosher). They never eat pork. Some hospitals store deep-frozen Kosher meals.

The local Jewish community usually organizes a group of people to care for patients in hospital. Most families want to be present at the moment of death. Some members of the family or the community may wish to remain in the hospital with the body after death.

After death, it is advisable to wear disposable gloves so that there is no direct contact with the body. Members of the Jewish community will probably wash and prepare the body for burial. No mutilation of the body is allowed unless an autopsy is required for legal reasons. The funeral is usually held within 24 hours.

Relatives are encouraged to express their grief openly – three days of intense grief, followed by grieving periods of seven days and 30 days for re-adjustment. The Jewish community is very supportive during this time.

Islam

Islam is the Arabic word for submission, surrender, obedience. 'There is no God but Allah.' Mohammed is the prophet sent by God. Muslims come from all over the world. In the UK, most are from India, Bangladesh, Pakistan, North Africa and Arab countries.

The *Qur'an* is the Holy Book revealed to the prophet Mohammed. The five pillars of Islam are

- there is only one God
- prayers five times a day
- almsgiving
- fasting
- pilgrimage to Mecca.

Islam does not have an organized ministry comparable to the Christian clergy. There is respect for 'holy men' (imams), which could include hospital chaplains. Friday is the Holy Day.

Other features include

- diet – pork and alcohol are forbidden, some are vegetarian
- modesty – the women are reluctant to undress for examination
- cleanliness – great importance attached to personal hygiene
- prayer – facing Mecca, i.e. south-east.

When dying, friends may read from the *Qur'an* and whisper the Muslim articles of faith in order to bring peace to the soul.[17]

The body should not be touched by the hospital staff. Disposable gloves should be used for the Last Offices. The head should be turned to the right before rigor mortis sets in. Family members of the same sex as the deceased may attend to the washing of the body. The body is buried as quickly as possible. Autopsy is allowed only if legally necessary. Cremation is prohibited; coffins are not used.

Many Asian people with their close-knit families find it difficult to accept our Western idea of restricted visiting. The whole family feel bound to visit as often as possible.

Hinduism

Hinduism dates back to about 2500 BC. There is no single prophet, no formal creed or central authority.

Worship is often in the home. Even in a temple there is no set pattern of worship. There is a complex system of gods and goddesses who are subsidiary to the Supreme Being. The guru (teacher, guide) occupies an important place in guiding the Hindu on his path through life.

Beliefs include transmigration of the soul with an indefinite number of re-incarnations until the attainment of Nirvana or fusion with the Supreme Being.

Other features include

- names – personal name, complementary name, and family name
- diet – the cow is sacred and Hindus are forbidden to eat beef. Many Hindus are vegetarian
- modesty – many Asian women find undressing embarrassing
- cleanliness – prefer to wash in running water. The left hand is used for unclean tasks, e.g. toilet; the right hand for clean tasks, e.g. eating.

When a Hindu is dying, a Hindu priest should be contacted if the family wish it. Relatives often go home and do not stay at the bedside.[18]

A Hindu prefers to die at home, preferably on the floor near Mother Earth. He may want to do this in hospital. The relatives should be asked about washing the body etc. They may want to do this and put on new clothes. Autopsy is not forbidden but is considered distasteful. Cremation is usual.

Sikhism

Founded in the fifteenth century AD, Sikhism is a society in which every member works for the common good. 'Sikh' means 'disciple'. Most come from the Punjab.

Teaches that everyone should have a direct communication with God, and that none should have special privileges by reason of birth, wealth, religion, race or sex. The way of salvation is through a good life of kindness to others and concern for family and society. Belief in re-incarnation. Women have equal status with men and are outgoing and ready to enter society. There are no priests in Sikhism.

A Sikh is identified by five marks, the removal of any of which would be distressing and offensive

- uncut hair and beard
- comb ('top knot' of hair) and turban
- steel bangle – reminder of the unity of God
- sword – now often worn as a brooch
- shorts – reminder of sexual discipline.

Other features include

- names – personal name, title Singh (lion) for men and Kaur (princess) for women, and family name
- diet – do not eat beef
- modesty – women prefer to be examined by a female doctor or to have a female chaperone
- prayers – appreciate privacy for personal prayers.

When close to death the relevant part of the Sikh scriptures are read. Sikh hymns are read over the dead body in the home. There is no objection to staff handling the body. Cremation is favoured; ashes are thrown into water.

Buddhism

Buddhism arose against a background of Hinduism in the sixth century BC. Buddha is not revered as a god, but as an example of a way of life. Buddhahood must be realized within ourselves through prayer and virtuous conduct.

Belief in re-incarnation. Accept responsibility for their lives because the consequences of present actions will have an effect on future lives, until Nirvana is attained where individuals lose identity and merge with the Supreme Being. Buddhists may appreciate a time of peace and quiet for meditation to help achieve inner calm. Buddhism condemns contraceptives, abortion, euthanasia. It accepts blood transfusion and transplants. No foods are forbidden, but some Buddhists are vegetarian.

Helping people is fundamental to the Buddhist ideal and the patient will always respect those (doctor, nurse, etc.) helping him. The family should be consulted whenever possible about specific wishes or needs. It may be possible to contact a local Buddhist priest when a Buddhist patient is dying.

A dying Buddhist may wish to maintain clarity of thought as long as possible and may decline analgesics if these induce somnolence.[19] There are no specific rituals related to Last Offices; anyone may prepare the body. Cremation is usual. White is the colour of mourning.

Bereavement
(Marilyn Relf)

> '"Mourning [grieving] is not forgetting" he said gently, his helplessness vanishing and his voice becoming wise. "It is an undoing. Every minute tie has to be untied and something permanent and valuable recovered and assimilated from the knot. The end is gain, of course. Blessed are they that mourn [grieve], for they shall be made strong. But the process is like all other human births, painful and long and dangerous."[20]
>
> 'An affliction of the heart may be physical as well as spiritual. Always it is the whole person who must be healed. For what hurts one part hurts the whole.'[21]

People often think of grief as an emotional experience. It is – but it is also a physical, intellectual, social and spiritual experience.[22] Grief not only affects how a person feels, it also affects behaviour. Some of the many and varied reactions are listed below (Table 2.1). Note how grief may lead to apathy in some but overactivity in others – or both in the same person at different times.

The process of grief

Personal crises

- provide new insights
- change one's understanding of the world
- have a major formative impact.

Table 2.1: Common reactions to grief

Physical reactions	
Sighing	Weakness and fatigue
Tachycardia	Increased blood pressure
Muscular tension	Sleep disturbances
Decreased resistance to illness	Weight and appetite change
	Increased sensory awareness
Self-neglect	
Emotional reactions	
Numbness	Anger
Sadness	Spiritual connectedness
Despair	Euphoria
Feeling of being lost	Yearning
Peacefulness	Helplessness
Confusion	Bitterness
Guilt	Vengefulness
Hopelessness	Relief
Behavioural reactions	
Searching	Decreased activity/apathetic
Disorientation	Detached from surroundings
Poor concentration	Withdrawn from friends and activities
Blaming others	
Pre-occupied	Forgetful
Seeking solitude	Crying
	Increased activity

Bereavement is the greatest personal crisis which many people ever have to face. Grief is a transitional process.[23] By grieving, the bereaved person adjusts to the loss and the meaning of that loss in her life. In other words, the reality of an external event is assimilated internally.

In the UK, changes in society over the last 50 years have affected the way loss and bereavement are perceived

- people expect to live longer and be healthier because of improved health care, e.g. antibiotics, better nutrition and the absence of war
- people commonly do not experience bereavement before adulthood because of decreased infant and child mortality
- families are smaller and more scattered
- people live in smaller units.

The bereaved, particularly the elderly, feel more isolated and turn to professionals (notably the general practitioner) or to support groups (such as Cruse) for help and understanding. Many people do not easily seek help. This increases the feeling of isolation experienced by the bereaved.

The process of grief has been described in several different models

- phases of grief[23]
- tasks of mourning[24]
- dimensions of loss.[25]

Phases of grief

Shock, numbness and disbelief

Initially, bereaved people may feel as if they are detached from reality. Because the reality of the death has not yet fully penetrated awareness, they may appear outwardly to have accepted the loss.

Separation and pain

'The absence of the dead person is everywhere palpable. The home and family environs seem full of painful reminders. Grief breaks over the bereaved in waves of distress. There is intense yearning, as if the dead person has been torn out of his body.'[23]

Shock and numbness gradually gives way to intense feelings.

Searching behaviour is common

- 'seeing' the dead person in the street
- other misinterpretations, including hallucinations
- dreaming about the deceased
- revisiting favourite places in the hope that the deceased might be there.

Despair

Despair sets in when it is realized that the lost person will not return. Poor concentration, anger, guilt, irritability, anxiety, restlessness and extreme sadness become common.

Acceptance

Bereaved people may be intellectually aware of the finality of the loss long before their emotions let them accept the truth. Depression and emotional swings may continue for more than a year after bereavement. Despair gradually gives way to acceptance of the loss.

Resolution and re-organization

As old patterns of life are given up, new patterns without the dead person are adopted and the bereaved person enters the phase of resolution or re-organization. Eventually the bereaved person is able to remember the deceased without being overwhelmed by sadness or other emotions and is ready to re-invest in the world.

This model implies a certain passivity. It is limited because it suggests that bereavement proceeds from one clearly identifiable reaction to another in an orderly fashion. This is not the case. The model should be used with care to avoid inappropriate behaviour towards bereaved people, such as hasty judgements of where individuals are or ought to be in their grief.

Tasks of mourning

The process of grief has also been described as a series of tasks to be completed by the bereaved in order to move towards resolution

- accept the reality of the loss
- experience the pain of grief
- adjust to an environment in which the dead person is missing
- withdraw emotional energy and re-invest in other relationships/ activities.

By encouraging the bereaved to work through the tasks of mourning, it is possible to facilitate the process of grief. The thought that something can be done and there is an end point is a powerful antidote to the feelings of helplessness experienced by most bereaved persons.

Dimensions of loss

This model focuses on how loss affects all the dimensions of life. It emphasizes that loss demands many adjustments, some of which are likely to be easier than others.

Identity

- how far has a person been able to accept the loss:
  intellectually?
  emotionally?
- how has it changed the person's concept of themselves and how has it affected self-esteem?

Emotional

- how freely is the person able to express emotions?
- how much has the person's emotional equilibrium been affected?

Spiritual

- what meaning has the bereaved ascribed to the experience?
- how has it affected religious beliefs, personal philosophy and the inner spiritual 'core'?

Practical

- is the person able to deal with the day-to-day practicalities of life such as cooking, shopping, looking after himself and the home?

Physical

- how has the bereaved person's health been affected:
  having trouble sleeping?
  losing weight?
  experiencing stress-related symptoms?

Lifestyle

- has the bereaved person's lifestyle had to change?
- will she have to move house, start work, deal with finances?

Family and community

- how has the person's role changed:
  within the family, e.g. by taking on the deceased person's role
    as a mother or father?
  within society, e.g. what does it mean to be a widow rather than
    a wife?
- do friends treat the bereaved person differently?
- how isolated is the bereaved person?

Understanding the phases of grief, the tasks of mourning and the dimensions of loss helps one to understand the impact of bereavement on an individual.

Sources of help

In addition to the clergy, general practitioner, district nurse and social worker, there are two main organizations in the UK which offer help in bereavement or give advice.

Cruse
126 Sheen Road, Richmond, Surrey TW9 1UR
Tel: 0181 940 4818/9047

Cruse offers support to all bereaved people, both counselling and social activities. It has about 200 branches in the UK.

National Association of Bereavement Services
20 Norton Folgate, London E1 6DB
Tel: 0171 247 1080/0617

This is an umbrella organization for local bereavement services. It publishes a national directory of bereavement services.

Risk assessment in bereavement

'Statistical studies confirm that secure people whose experience of life has led to a reasonable trust in themselves and others will cope well with anticipated bereavements, provided they are well supported by a family who respects their need to grieve. However, multiple or unexpected and untimely losses of people on whom one depends or who depended on the survivor can overwhelm the most secure person, and lack of security and support can undermine a person's capacity to cope.'[26]

People vary in their response to bereavement. Grief may be

- immediate or delayed
- brief or seem unending
- severe or mild.

Most people work through their grief with the help of family and friends. Some report that they feel stronger and more mature. A significant minority suffer prolonged impairment of their physical and psychological health. Bereavement is associated with health risks. It

- predisposes people to physical and mental illness
- precipitates illness and death
- exacerbates existing illness
- leads to or exacerbates health threatening behaviour such as smoking, drinking and drug use
- results in an increased use of health services
- may lead to depression.[27]

Several factors have been found to be associated with a good or poor outcome. These can be identified at the time of bereavement and can be used to focus resources in order to prevent or ameliorate 'complicated' grief.[26]

Mode of death

- was it timely or untimely?
- was it expected or unexpected?
- was it unduly disturbing for the relatives or key carers?

Deaths that are untimely, unexpected and/or unduly disturbing are likely to cause more severe and more prolonged grief. *The death of someone with terminal illness can still be unexpected.*

Nature of the relationship

How ambivalent was the relationship between the key carer and the patient? In a highly ambivalent relationship there is likely to be a more difficult bereavement. Often this manifests as persistent feelings of guilt.

How necessary was the deceased for the key carer's sense of well-being, self-esteem or security? The more dependent the relationship the more all pervading the sense of loss.

Perceived support

- is the bereaved person able to share her feelings with family and friends?
- does she feel supported or isolated in her loss?

Anticipatory grieving

- were the family and patient able to talk about the illness, share feelings, and make plans for the future before the patient died?

Periods of denial by both patient and family are normal during a terminal illness but an excessive use of denial may make it harder for the survivor to start sharing with others after the patient's death.

Anger also may impede the process of grief. Angry people may deflect support and find themselves isolated.

Concurrent life events

- how much stress is the key carer/family currently facing?
  finances
  menopause
  children leaving home
  unemployment
  retirement
- how many people are dependent on the key carer, e.g. children or elderly relatives?
- has she time and space to grieve?

Previous losses

- how has the person grieved in the past?
- will the new loss uncover unresolved loss?

Medical history

- has the person a concurrent physical or psychological illness which is likely to be exacerbated by the loss?
- is there a history of alcoholism, drug abuse or suicidal behaviour?

The most positive factor in favour of a good outcome is the presence of a supportive family and/or friends who allow the bereaved person to express grief and to talk unconditionally about feelings for as long as is needed.[28]

Children and bereavement
(Ann Couldrick, Rosalyn Staveley)

About 2% of children under 16 in the UK have lost at least one parent by death. The death of the father comprises 80% of these parental deaths.

Studies suggest that children are most deeply affected not by the actual loss but by the

- significance of the relationship with the remaining parent
- emotional climate in which the child is helped to come to terms with the loss.

There are several severe disruptions and changes which may affect the child

- the bereaved spouse is grieving
- other adults may or may not take on the dead parent's function
- the child may not understand what has happened because he has not been given clear information
- there may be changes of home and of school
- the family may have fewer social contacts
- there may be social and economic decline particularly when the father dies
- the surviving parent may remarry before the child has fully understood the dead parent is not going to return
- the child may be taken into care.

The majority of bereaved children do adjust normally, and in time are less disturbed than children in families where there is severe marital discord.

Adults frequently do not know what to expect and may deny that a child is affected. They are often unable to perceive or respond to the very clear signals of the child's distress. This is related to the adult's own way of dealing with the loss, which may be pathological.

The effect of bereavement on children

Physical responses

- sleep disturbances, e.g. insomnia, bad dreams
- eating disorders, e.g. loss of appetite, compulsive eating, craving certain foods

- toileting difficulties, e.g. children previously continent who start to wet and soil are signalling distress
- physical symptoms may occur, e.g. rashes, fever, nausea, or existing conditions exacerbated, e.g. asthma, eczema. In an older child, symptoms frequently mimic those of the person who has died.

Emotional responses

- increased generalized anxiety often resulting in the child not wanting to leave home or go to school
- becoming more clinging and dependent
- exaggerated separation responses, e.g. intense distress when the carer walks out of the room or leaves for short periods
- rapid mood swings from euphoric and all right to weeping, depression, rejection of carer(s), withdrawal, or inappropriately aggressive responses in various situations.

Cognitive effects

- poor concentration
- loss of short term and/or long term memory
- poor or changed motivation, e.g. 'What is the point of anything now?'
- learning difficulties, e.g. an existing undiagnosed problem may become evident or a new difficulty may develop, the nature of which will depend upon the child's developmental stage.

Behavioural responses

- an obvious anxiety about or dislike of change in routine(s)
- regression to infant needs, e.g. wanting to be fed, rocked in parent's arms

- 'acting out' behaviour reflecting an unconscious and often aggress-ive response which seems unrelated to feelings and needs, e.g. playing very loud music, dangerous competitive activities such as racing bikes or cars, and stealing
- putting on a 'brave face' for the sake of the surviving parent, or because of a fear of losing control.

Approach the parent as a colleague

Remember, parents have expert knowledge about their children. Boost confidence and increase their feelings of competence by

- explaining the physical, emotional, cognitive and behavioural changes which might occur and re-assure parents that these are normal reactions for children
- recommending appropriate books and leaflets. These help some parents to gain intellectual mastery over the situation. Books to read with children can be important as a less direct way of approaching a discussion
- suggesting that parents encourage children to draw, paint or write about their experience of the loss and to talk about the implications if they wish to
- suggesting that the children are encouraged to make a scrapbook of memories, e.g. photos, cards, letters, and collecting mementos and talking about these
- warning parents that children's play and interests may appear to revolve around dying, death and funerals. This is a natural way for children to work through their difficulties and gain a greater understanding of the world
- telling parents not to be too hard on themselves. It is normal sometimes to shout or be impatient with children – parents need only to be 'good enough'

- giving parents 'permission' to be open with the children about how they are feeling themselves. In doing this, parents are modelling the honest expression of feelings:
  'I'm crying because I am sad'
  'I'm angry because we cannot do that together again'
  'I'm laughing because I am remembering how funny it was when . . .'

- encouraging parents to involve others (relatives, friends, teachers) for both practical help and emotional support

- being aware of and sensitive to the family belief and value systems – go along with their beliefs and values and do not impose your own – avoid 'ought' and 'should'

- encouraging parents to look after their own physical, practical and emotional needs. If they do, parents will be better able to deal with the children's needs and demands.

PART THREE

Symptom
Management I

General principles · Pain
Pain in advanced cancer
Pain management · Nonopioids
Weak opioids · Strong opioids
Neuropathic pain · Useful definitions

General principles

The scientific approach to pain and symptom management can be
summarized as

- evaluation
- explanation
- individualized treatment
- supervision
- attention to detail.

Patients are often reluctant to bother their doctor about minor symptoms such as dry mouth, altered taste, anorexia, pruritus, cough and insomnia. Enquiries should be made from time to time rather than rely on spontaneous reports.

Evaluation

Evaluation must precede treatment

The cancer itself is not always the cause of a symptom. Further, some symptoms are caused by several factors. Causal factors include

- cancer
- treatment
- debility
- concurrent disorder.

Treatment depends on the underlying pathological mechanism

Even when the cancer is responsible, a symptom may be caused in different ways, e.g. vomiting from hypercalcaemia and vomiting from raised intracranial pressure. Treatment will vary accordingly.

Explanation

Explain the underlying mechanism(s) in simple terms

Treatment begins with an explanation by the doctor of the reason(s) for the symptom. This knowledge does much to reduce the psychological impact of the symptom on the sufferer:

> 'The shortness of breath is caused partly by the cancer itself and partly by fluid at the base of the right lung. In addition, you are anaemic.'

If explanation is omitted, the patient may continue to think that his condition is shrouded in mystery. This is frightening because 'even the doctors don't know what's going on'.

Individualized treatment

Do not limit treatment to the use of drugs

- treatment may be physical or psychological or both
- treatment may be drug or nondrug or both.

For example, pruritus is relieved in the majority of patients without resort to antihistamines. Aqueous cream applied to dry, itching skin several times a day, and soap eliminated in favour of emulsifying ointment is frequently sufficient.

Prescribe drugs prophylactically for persistent symptoms

When treating a persistent symptom with a drug, it should be administered regularly on a prophylactic basis. The use of drugs 'as needed' instead of regularly is the cause of much unrelieved distress.

Keep the treatment as simple as possible

When an additional drug is considered, ask the following questions:

'What is the treatment goal?'

'How can it be monitored?'

'What is the risk of adverse effects?'

'What is the risk of drug interactions?'

'Is it possible to stop any of the current medication?'

Never say 'I have tried everything' or 'There is nothing more I can do'

It is generally possible to develop a repertoire of alternative measures. Although it is wise not to promise too much, it is important to re-assure the patient that you are going to stand by him and do all you can to help, e.g. 'No promises but we'll do our best.'

Instead of attempting immediately to relieve a symptom completely, be prepared to chip away at the problem a little at a time. When tackled in this way it is surprising how much can be achieved with determination and persistence.

Written advice is essential

Precise guidelines are necessary to achieve maximum patient co-operation. 'Take as much as you like, as often as you like' is a recipe for anxiety, poor symptom relief and maximum adverse effects. The drug regimen should be written out in full for the patient and his family to work from. Time to be taken, names of drugs, reason for use (for pain, for bowels, etc.) and dose (x ml, y tablets) should all be stated. Also there should be details of what to do when medication runs out.

Supervision

Review! Review! Review!

It is often difficult to predict the optimum dose of a symptom relief drug, particularly opioids, laxatives and psychotropic drugs. Further, adverse effects put drug compliance in jeopardy. Arrangements must be made for continuing supervision and adjustment of medication.

It is sometimes necessary to compromise on complete relief in order to avoid unacceptable adverse effects. For example, anticholinergic effects such as dry mouth or visual disturbance may limit dose escalation. With inoperable bowel obstruction it may be better to aim to reduce the incidence of vomiting to once or twice a day rather than to seek complete relief.

Cancer is a progressive disease, and new symptoms occur. These must be dealt with urgently.

Attention to detail

Attention to detail requires an inquisitive mind, one which repeatedly asks why:

> 'Thou shalt not make assumptions.'
>
> 'To *ass-u-me* is to make an *ass* of *u* and *me*.'[29]

'Why is this patient with breast cancer vomiting? She is not taking morphine; she is not hypercalcaemic. Why is she vomiting?'

'This patient with cancer of the pancreas has pain in the neck. It does not fit with the usual pattern of metastatic spread. Why does he have pain there?'

Attention to detail is important at every stage – in evaluation, explanation (e.g. avoid jargon; use simple language) and when planning and prescribing treatment (e.g. preparing written advice and drug regimens which are easy to follow).

Attention to detail makes all the difference to palliative care – without it success may be forfeited and patients suffer needlessly.

Pain

'Pain is what the patient says hurts.'

Pain is an unpleasant *sensory* and *emotional* experience associated with actual or potential tissue damage or described in terms of such damage.[30] In other words, pain is a *somatopsychic* phenomenom. The perception of pain is modulated by

- the patient's *mood*
- the patient's *morale*
- the *meaning* of the pain for the patient.

The meaning of persistent pain in advanced cancer is 'I am incurable, I am going to die'. Other factors affecting pain threshold are shown in Table 3.1. Because of the multidimensional nature of pain, it is often

Table 3.1:   Factors affecting pain threshold

Threshold lowered	Threshold raised
Discomfort	Relief of other symptoms
Insomnia	Sleep
Fatigue	Sympathy
Anxiety	Understanding
Fear	Companionship
Anger	Creative activity
Sadness	Relaxation
Depression	Reduction in anxiety/anxiolytics
Boredom	
Mental isolation	Elevation of mood/antidepressants
Social abandonment	
	Analgesics

helpful to think in terms of 'total pain', encompassing the physical, psychological, social and spiritual aspects of suffering.

People suffering from chronic pain usually do not look in pain because of the absence of autonomic concomitants (Table 3.2). In cancer, acute pain concomitants may be evident particularly if the pain is severe and of recent onset or paroxysmal.

Because of the implications for treatment, it is also important to distinguish between pain caused by stimulation of nerve endings (nociceptive pain) and pain caused by nerve dysfunction (neuropathic pain). Neuropathic pain is often only partially responsive to treatment with standard analgesics, including morphine and other opioids

Table 3.2: Temporal classification of pain

	Acute	Chronic	
Time course	Transient	Persistent	
Meaning to patient	Positive draws attention to injury or illness	Negative serves no useful purpose	Positive as patient obtains second- ary gain
Concomitants	Fight or flight pupillary dilatation increased sweating tachypnoea tachycardia shunting of blood from viscera to muscles	Vegetative sleep disturbance anorexia decreased libido no pleasure in life constipation somatic pre- occupation personality change lethargy	

Table 3.3: Types of pain and implications for treatment

Type of pain	Mechanism	Example	Response to opioids	Treatment
Nociceptive				
visceral	Stimulation of nerve endings	Hepatic capsule pain	+	Analgesics
somatic		Bone pain	+/–	Analgesics
muscle spasm			–	Muscle relaxant
Neuropathic				
nerve compression	Stimulation of nervi nervorum (?)		+/–	Analgesics; corticosteroid
neural injury	Peripheral nerve injury ('de-afferentation pain')	Neuroma or nerve infiltration (e.g. brachial or lumbo-sacral plexus)	(+)/–	Trial of opioid; trial of corticosteroid; tricyclic antidepressant; anticonvulsant; local anaesthetic congener; spinal analgesia; ketamine; TENS
	CNS injury	Spinal cord compression or post-stroke pain		
sympathetically-mediated	Abnormal sympathetic activity	Causalgia	–	Sympathetic nerve block

(*see* p.93). Thus, from a therapeutic point of view, it is often helpful to think of pain in cancer in terms of the response to opioids (Table 3.3):

Opioid responsive, i.e. pain relieved by opioids

Opioid semiresponsive, i.e. pain relieved by the concurrent use of an opioid and an adjuvant drug ('co-analgesic')

Opioid resistant, i.e. pain not relieved by opioids.

Opioid resistance may be more apparent than real (Table 3.4). Painful muscle spasm (cramp) is a good example of true opioid resistant pain.

Table 3.4: Opioid resistant cancer pain: clinical classification

Pseudoresistant
Underdosing
Poor alimentary absorption (*rare*)
Poor alimentary absorption because of vomiting
Ignoring psychological aspects of care
Semiresistant/semiresponsive
Soft tissue ⎫
Muscle infiltration ⎬ associated with local inflammation
Bone metastasis ⎭
Neuropathic (some)
Raised intracranial pressure
Activity related
Resistant
Neuropathic (some)
Muscle spasm

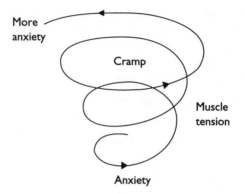

Figure 3.1:   Relationship between anxiety and cramp.

Cramp in various parts of the body is relatively common in cancer. It is often associated with bone pain exacerbated by movement. Anxiety is a potent exacerbating factor (Figure 3.1).

Myofascial pain is a specific form of cramp. Myofascial trigger points occur most commonly in the pectoral girdle and neck.

Pain in advanced cancer

Pain and advanced cancer are not synonymous

- three quarters of patients experience pain
- one quarter of patients do not experience pain.

Multiple concurrent pains are common in those who have pain

- one fifth have one pain
- four fifths have two or more pains
- one third have four or more pains.

Pain in cancer can be grouped into four causal categories

- caused by cancer itself
- caused by treatment
- related to cancer and/or debility
- caused by a concurrent disorder.

Individual common causes in a group of patients with advanced cancer are shown below (Table 3.5).

Table 3.5: Top ten pains in patients with advanced cancer at Sobell House ($n = 211$)

1 Bone	
2 Visceral	caused by cancer itself
3 Neuropathic	
4 Soft tissue	
5 Immobility	
6 Constipation	
7 Myofascial	related to cancer and/or debility
8 Cramp	
9 Oesophagitis	
10 Degeneration of the spine	concurrent disorder

Pain management

Pain relief may be achieved by one or more of the following methods.

Examination

- to establish trust
- to confirm site
- to identify cause.

Explanation

- to reduce psychological impact of pain.

Modification of pathological process

- radiation therapy
- hormone therapy
- chemotherapy
- surgery.

Elevation of pain threshold

- nondrug methods (*see* Table 3.1, p.68)
- primary analgesics
- secondary analgesics
- psychotropic drugs.

Interruption of pain pathways

● local anaesthesia:
  lignocaine
  bupivacaine

● neurolysis:
  chemical (alcohol, phenol)
  cold (cryotherapy)
  heat (thermocoagulation)

● neurosurgery:
  coeliac axis plexus block
  intrathecal phenol
  cervical spinothalamic tractotomy (cordotomy).

Modification of way of life and environment

● avoid pain-precipitating activities

● immobilization of painful part:
  cervical collar
  surgical corset
  slings
  orthopaedic surgery

● walking aid

● wheelchair

● hoist.

If anticancer treatment is recommended, analgesics should also be given until the treatment ameliorates the pain – which may take several weeks in the case of chemotherapy. Sometimes, satisfactory results are obtained only be combining several treatments. The use of analgesics is one way of elevating the patient's pain threshold, thereby reducing perception of pain.

Since the advent of spinal analgesia (*see* p.98), neurolytic and neurosurgical procedures have become relatively obsolete. At many centres, coeliac axis plexus block with alcohol for epigastric visceral pain is the only neurolytic block which is still used.

Some patients continue to experience pain on movement despite analgesics, other drugs, radiotherapy and nerve blocks. Here, the situation is often improved by suggesting modifications to the patient's way of life and environment (*see previous page*). This is where the help of a physiotherapist and an occupational therapist is often invaluable.

It is generally best to aim at 'graded' pain relief

- relief at night
- relief at rest during the day
- relief on movement (not always completely possible).

Relief should be evaluated in relation to each pain. If there is severe anxiety and/or depression, it may take three to four weeks to achieve maximum benefit. Re-evaluation is a continuing necessity; old pains may get worse and new ones develop.

Principles of analgesic use

For pain caused by the cancer itself, drugs usually give adequate relief provided the right drug is administered in the right dose at the right time intervals.

By the mouth

The oral route is the preferred route for analgesics, including morphine and other strong opioids.

By the clock

Persistent pain requires preventive therapy. This means that analgesics should be given regularly and prophylactically. 'As needed' medication is irrational and inhumane.

By the ladder

Use a three-step analgesic ladder (Figure 3.2). If a drug fails to relieve, *move up the ladder*; do not move laterally in the same efficacy group.

Individual treatment

The right dose of an analgesic is the dose which relieves the pain.

Supervision

The response to treatment must be monitored to ensure that benefits of treatment are maximized and adverse effects minimized.

Adjuvant drugs

A laxative is almost always necessary with an opioid; about 50% of patients need an anti-emetic (Table 3.6).

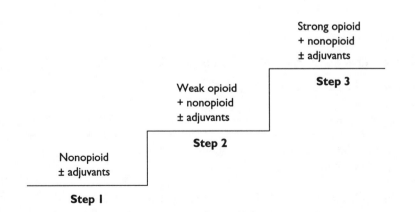

Figure 3.2:   The World Health Organization 3-step analgesic ladder.[31]

Table 3.6: Adjuvant drugs for analgesic ladder

Control of adverse effects

Laxative

Anti-emetic

Psychotropic medication

Night sedative

Anxiolytic

Antidepressant

Co-analgesic

Corticosteroid

Nonopioids

The main nonopioids are

- aspirin
- other nonsteroidal anti-inflammatory drugs (NSAIDs)
- paracetamol/acetaminophen.

Nonopioids are step 1 analgesics. Because of their anti-inflammatory effect, NSAIDs are particularly useful for metastatic bone and soft tissue pains. In these circumstances, they should be used even when a strong opioid is also necessary.

In hot countries, NSAIDs are sometimes discouraged because of the risk of acute renal failure in hypovolaemic patients. Paracetamol is used instead.

Mode of action

Nonopioids inhibit prostaglandin (PG) synthesis by inhibiting the enzyme cyclo-oxygenase. They do this to a variable extent in different tissues. For example, paracetamol inhibits PG synthesis in the *brain* but has no effect on PG synthesis in inflamed joints. Thus, although paracetamol is analgesic and antipyretic (like the NSAIDs), it manifests no anti-inflammatory properties in rheumatoid arthritis. Sulindac also shows clear selectivity; unlike other NSAIDs it has no effect on renal PG synthesis.

The relative benefits of the NSAIDs and paracetamol in painful bone metastases have yet to be determined. Likewise, the extent of the central analgesic effect of most NSAIDs is unknown.

Inhibition of PG synthesis does not account for the total analgesic effect of NSAIDs, although it appears to explain most of the adverse effects. In postdental extraction pain, most weak inhibitors of cyclo-oxygenase are significantly superior to aspirin and most strong inhibitors are inferior. Ketorolac is an example of a weak cyclo-oxygenase inhibitor which is superior to aspirin and most other NSAIDs in terms of analgesic efficacy.

Nonopioids and platelet function

- aspirin causes *irreversible* impairment of platelet function (with prolongation of bleeding time) by inactivating platelet cyclo-oxygenase permanently by acetylation

- most other NSAIDs cause reversible impairment of platelet function

- *nonacetylated salicylates* have no effect on platelet function at normal therapeutic doses:
    choline magnesium salicylate
    diflunisal
    salsalate.

Common adverse effects and interactions

- gastric erosions, peptic ulcers, haemorrhage:
    more with cheap standard aspirin tablets because of coarse granular nature

    less with dispersible and enteric-coated aspirin, comparable to other NSAIDs

    ibuprofen (available 'over the counter') is least toxic in this respect

- many NSAIDs can induce bronchospasm in susceptible patients:
    paracetamol also causes bronchospasm in about 25% of aspirin sensitive patients

    choline salicylate, choline magnesium trisalicylate, azapropazone and benzydamine do not cause bronchospasm

- aspirin may cause tinnitus and deafness, particularly in hypoalbuminaemic patients

- all NSAIDs cause salt and water retention which may result in ankle oedema. In consequence, they *antagonize* the action of diuretics to a variable extent

- aspirin *potentiates* oral hypoglycaemic agents

- aspirin *antagonizes* uricosuric agents.

Distinguishing features of paracetamol

- it usually can be taken by those hypersensitive to aspirin

- it does not injure the gastric mucosa

- it is well tolerated by patients with peptic ulcers

- it does not affect plasma uric acid concentration

- it has no effect on platelet function

- liquid preparations are stable

- adverse effects are unusual.

The main drawback with paracetamol is the frequency of administration (q4h–q6h). Because NSAIDs are mainly peripheral in action and paracetamol central, the two can be used in combination with an additive effect.

Choice of NSAID

This depends on several factors, e.g. availability, fashion, cost, frequency of administration, individual toxicity and response. Typical regimens include:

Ibuprofen	400–600 mg q.d.s.
Flurbiprofen	50–100 mg b.d.
Naproxen	250–500 mg b.d.
Diflunisal	250–500 mg b.d.
Diclofenac (m/r)	100–200 mg o.d.
Benorylate suspension	5–10 ml b.d.

Weak opioids

Weak opioids in combination with nonopioids are step 2 analgesics (Table 3.7). A weak opioid is as effective as a small dose of morphine. This means that step 2 is pharmacologically unnecessary. In many countries, however, it is much easier to obtain and supply a weak opioid preparation.

Codeine is a prodrug of morphine. It is about 1/10 as potent as morphine. *About 10% of the population cannot convert codeine to morphine.* A typical dose range for codeine is 30–60 mg q4h. In the UK, dihydrocodeine is generally used instead.

Table 3.7: Commonly used weak opioid compound preparations (UK)

Generic name		Drug content	
		Weak opioid	Nonopioid
Co-codaprin	8/400	Codeine 8 mg	Aspirin 400 mg
Co-codamol	8/500	Codeine 8 mg	Paracetamol 500 mg
Co-codamol	30/500	Codeine 30 mg	Paracetamol 500 mg
Co-dydramol	10/500	Dihydrocodeine 10 mg	Paracetamol 500 mg
Co-proxamol	32.5/325	Dextropropoxy- phene hydro- chloride 32.5 mg	Paracetamol 325 mg

Tramadol

Tramadol is an alternative opioid for both step 2 and the lower end of step 3. Its exact relative potency with oral codeine and oral morphine in cancer patients is still debatable. By injection, it is 1/10 as potent as morphine. In Table 3.8 (*see* p.89) it is regarded as double strength codeine, i.e. 1/5 strength morphine. This difference relates to the high oral bio-availability of tramadol (about 70%).

Tramadol has a dual mechanism of analgesic action, part opioid and part a presynaptic re-uptake blocker of mono-amines (like a tricyclic antidepressant; *see* p.100). It does not have anticholinergic or anti-depressant properties. The dual analgesic action is synergistic. Un-wanted opioid effects are significantly less than with codeine and morphine.

Strong opioids

These are step 3 analgesics. As in step 2, a nonopioid should normally be given concurrently.

Morphine and other strong opioids exist to be given, not merely to be withheld. Their use is dictated by therapeutic need, not by brevity of prognosis.

Morphine does not cause clinically important respiratory depression in cancer patients in pain. This is because *pain is a physiological antagonist to the central depressant effects of morphine.* Further, in contrast to postoperative patients, cancer patients with pain:

- have usually been receiving a weak opioid for some time, i.e. are not opioid naive
- take medication by mouth (slower absorption, lower peak concentration)
- titrate the dose upwards step by step (less likelihood of an excessive 'standard' dose being given).

The relationship of the therapeutic dose to the lethal dose of morphine (the 'therapeutic ratio') is greater than commonly supposed. Patients who take a double dose of morphine at bedtime (see p.84) are no more likely to die during the night than those who do not.

Morphine is metabolized mainly to morphine-3-glucuronide and morphine-6-glucuronide. The former is inactive; the latter is a *more* potent analgesic than morphine itself. Both glucuronides cumulate in renal failure. This results in a prolonged duration of action for morphine, with danger of severe sedation and subsequent respiratory depression if the dose and/or frequency of administration are not reduced.

Tolerance to morphine is not a practical problem. Psychological dependence (addiction) does not occur if morphine is used correctly.

Physical dependence does not prevent a reduction in the dose of morphine if the patient's pain ameliorates, e.g. as a result of radio-therapy or a nerve block.

Morphine is not the panacea for cancer pain. Its use does not guarantee success, particularly if the psychosocial aspects of care are ignored.

Oral morphine

Morphine by mouth is the strong opioid of choice for cancer pain. It is administered as tablets (10 mg, 20 mg), in aqueous solutions (e.g. 2 mg in 1 ml), as m/r tablets (5 mg, 10 mg, 15 mg, 30 mg, 60 mg, 100 mg, 200 mg), or in a m/r suspension.

If previously receiving a weak opioid, begin with 10 mg q4h (m/r 30 mg q12h). With frail elderly patients, consider starting on 5 mg q4h in order to reduce initial drowsiness, confusion and unsteadiness.

If changing from an alternative strong opioid (e.g. buprenorphine, levorphanol, methadone) a much higher dose of morphine may be needed (*see* Table 3.8, p.89).

The patient should be advised to take additional 'as needed' doses between the regular doses if pain returns. Adjust the dose upwards after 24 hours if the pain is not 90% relieved (e.g. 5 to 10 mg, 10 to 15 mg, 20 to 30 mg).

Two thirds of patients never need more than 30 mg q4h (m/r morphine 100 mg q12h). The rest need up to 200 mg q4h (m/r morphine 600 mg q12h) and occasionally more.

> *With ordinary tablets or solution, a double dose at bedtime usually enables a patient to go through the night without waking in pain.*

Use adjuvants for bone pain (NSAID) and nerve compression pain (corticosteroid).

Supply an anti-emetic for regular use should nausea or vomiting develop, e.g. haloperidol 1.5 mg stat and nocte.

Prescribe a laxative, e.g. co-danthrusate. Adjust dose according to response. Suppositories and enemas continue to be necessary in about one third of patients. *Constipation may be more difficult to manage than the pain.*

Warn patients about the possibility of initial drowsiness.

Write out the drug regimen in detail with times, names of drugs and amount to be taken; arrange for follow-up.

If swallowing is difficult or vomiting persists, morphine may be given by suppository (same dose as PO). Alternatively, give half of the oral dose of morphine by SC injection or one third of the oral dose as SC diamorphine.

Diamorphine

Diamorphine hydrochloride (di-acetylmorphine, heroin) is available for medicinal use only in the UK and Canada. It is much more soluble than morphine sulphate/hydrochloride and is used in the UK instead of morphine when injections are necessary because large amounts can be given in very small volumes.

By injection, diamorphine is twice as potent as morphine. By this route, its initial effects are mediated by the primary metabolite, mono-acetylmorphine.

Because of rapid de-acetylation diamorphine by mouth is merely a prodrug for morphine. Possibly because of better absorption (it is highly lipid soluble), it is slightly more potent than morphine by this route.

Converting from morphine to diamorphine or changing routes

The following conversion ratios are approximate and should be regarded only as a general guide

- oral morphine to SC morphine, halve the oral dose
- oral morphine to IV morphine, give one third of the oral dose
- oral morphine to SC diamorphine, give one third of the oral dose
- oral diamorphine to SC diamorphine, halve the oral dose.

When changing from either oral diamorphine or oral morphine to m/r morphine, convert 1 mg for 1 mg and adjust as necessary.

There are no generic m/r morphine tablets. Because of differing pharmacokinetic profiles, it is best to keep individual patients on the same brand and not to change.

Morphine every four hours on general wards

Because most wards have only four drug rounds a day (0600, 1200, 1800 and 2200 h), special provision has to be made to enable a patient to receive morphine q4h. In practice, the interval between the first drug round (0600 h) and the last (2200 h) is usually less than 16 hours, and it is not uncommon to see a series of entries such as:

0725, 1125, 1550, 2130 h
0725, 1125, 1525, 1925, 2350 h

In the first example it proved impossible to give the third dose on time and the fourth has been delayed partly for convenience and partly to 'help you have a better night'. In the second example, the day staff have coped in an exemplary fashion with a highly individual regimen

– until bedtime, 'Here is your night sedative Mr Smith. You cannot have your morphine yet, it's not due. We'll bring it later'.

The patient either fails to get to sleep because of worry about the pain returning or complains bitterly when woken from a deep sleep by a nurse an hour or so later. In both instances, the comfort (and sleep) of the patient is put in jeopardy by a pharisaical attitude to the concept of 'every four hours'.

It is usually necessary to catch up at some stage in the day. Catching up is best done at 1000 h. If 'time slippage' occurs later in the day, catching up should be repeated, preferably at the next administration and certainly at 2200 h.

The interval between the early morning dose and the 1000 h dose is usually less than four hours, occasionally less than three. The nursing staff should be advised specifically on this point.

When catching up is practised, it is much easier for the nursing staff to administer medication every four hours. In fact, the only administration additional to the routine drug round is 1000 h. This is a time when the maximum number of nurses are available, and when Controlled Drug book-keeping is most easy to complete.

Check daily to ensure that all the prescribed doses have been given.

Most patients given a double dose at bedtime of ordinary morphine tablets or solution will sleep pain-free through the night.

Additional 'as needed' morphine should be prescribed for breakthrough pain. Instructions must be clear: the use of 'as needed' morphine does not mean that the next dose of regular morphine is omitted.

If 'as needed' morphine is requested several times a day, it is an indication that the regular dose needs to be adjusted upwards.

The availability of m/r tablets has simplified considerably the use of morphine on general wards.

Alternative strong opioids

There are multiple opioid receptor subtypes in many areas of the CNS, including the dorsal horn of the spinal cord. Mu, kappa and delta opioid receptors are all involved in analgesia. Opioids differ from each other in terms of intrinsic activity and receptor site affinity. This property can be utilized in patients who are intolerant of morphine (mainly a mu agonist) by converting, for example, to methadone (a mixed mu and delta agonist).

When converting from an alternative strong opioid to oral morphine, the initial dose depends on the relative potency of the two drugs (Table 3.8). Table 3.8 should also be used to determine an appropriate starting dose of an alternative opioid in someone intolerant of morphine (marked dysphoria and/or sedation, hallucinations, nausea and vomiting, pruritus which fail to respond to appropriate measures).

Pethidine and dextromoramide have little place in cancer pain management because of short durations of action. Some centres use dextromoramide for breakthrough pain in patients taking regular morphine, or as prophylactic additional analgesia before a painful dressing or other procedure. This is because of its rapid onset of action. Generally patients obtain satisfactory relief from an additional dose of morphine or by timing the procedure for one hour after a regular dose.

Pentazocine should not be used; it is a weak opioid by mouth and often causes psychotomimetic effects (dysphoria, depersonalization, frightening dreams, hallucinations).

Methadone

Methadone is a synthetic strong opioid. It is now widely regarded as the main alternative to morphine for cancer pain management. It has a broader spectrum of opioid receptor site affinities than morphine, and is useful in selected patients who experience poor relief and major adverse effects with morphine.

Table 3.8:   Approximate oral analgesic equivalence to morphine[a]

Analgesic	Potency ratio with morphine	Duration of action (hours)[b]
Codeine	1/10	3–5
Dihydrocodeine		
Pethidine (meperidine USA)	1/8	2–3
Tramadol	1/5	5–6
Dipipanone (in Diconal UK)	1/2	3–5
Papaveretum	2/3[c]	3–5
Oxycodone	4/3[d]	5–6
Dextromoramide	[2][e]	2–3
Methadone	[3–4][f]	6–12
Levorphanol	5	6–8
Phenazocine	5	6–8
Hydromorphone	8	3–5
Buprenorphine (*sublingual*)	60	6–8
Fentanyl (*transdermal*)	150	72

a   multiply dose of opioid by its potency ratio to determine the equivalent dose of morphine sulphate

b   dependent in part on severity of pain and on dose; often longer lasting in very elderly and those with renal dysfunction

c   papaveretum (strong opium) is standardized to contain 50% morphine base. Potency expressed in relation to morphine sulphate

d   oxycodone is three quarters as potent as morphine by injection but, because of greater oral bio-availability, it is more potent by mouth

e   dextromoramide: a single 5 mg dose is equivalent to morphine 15 mg in terms of peak effect but is shorter acting; overall potency ratio adjusted accordingly

f   methadone: a single 5 mg dose is equivalent to morphine 7.5 mg. Has a variable long plasma halflife which leads to cumulation in many patients; overall potency ratio adjusted accordingly

At Sobell House, methadone is used mainly in selected patients with renal failure who have developed excessive drowsiness and/or delirium with morphine because of cumulation of morphine-6-glucuronide. Methadone does not have a comparable active metabolite and its effects are therefore not altered in renal failure.

The plasma halflife of methadone ranges from 8–80 h. Cumulation is a potential problem for most patients. Dose titration is therefore different from morphine. After an initial 'run in' period when methadone is taken *q3h as needed*, most patients can be converted to b.d. or t.d.s.

Fentanyl

Fentanyl, like morphine, is mainly a strong mu agonist. It is widely used as a peri-operative analgesic. Transdermal patches (TTS-fentanyl) are available for cancer pain management. These deliver 25, 50, 75 or 100 mcg/h over three days. Peak plasma concentrations of fentanyl are achieved after 12–24 h and a depot remains in the skin for some 24 h after the patch is removed. A few patients obtain relief, however, for only 48 h rather than the intended 72 h. A conversion table for oral morphine to transdermal fentanyl is available. Patients who have not previously taken morphine or other strong opioid should start on the lowest dose, i.e. 25 mcg/h.

The patches do not permit rapid dose titration because of the slow onset of activity after application. Rescue medication will be necessary during the first 24 h. High fever and exposure of transdermal patches to external heat sources (e.g. heat pads, electric blankets) may increase the rate of delivery of fentanyl. There are considerable interpatient differences in the rate of metabolism and excretion of fentanyl.

Buprenorphine

Buprenorphine is a potent semisynthetic partial mu agonist. It is an alternative to oral morphine in the low to middle part of morphine's dose range.

In low doses, buprenorphine and morphine are additive in their effects; at very high doses, antagonism by buprenorphine may occur. There is no need, however, to prescribe both. Use one or the other; then unintended antagonism cannot occur.

Buprenorphine is available as a *sublingual* tablet; ingestion reduces bio-availability. It needs to be given only q8h. More frequent administration makes life unnecessarily harder for a hard-pressed patient. With daily doses of over 3 mg, patients may prefer to take fewer tablets q6h.

It is generally considered that there is an analgesic ceiling at a daily dose of 3–5 mg; equivalent to 180–300 mg of oral morphine/24 h. In some countries, 1.6 mg is regarded as the ceiling daily dose. Whether this represents genetic differences or local custom is not clear.

Buprenorphine is *not* an alternative to codeine or other weak opioid. Like morphine, it should be used when a weak opioid has failed. Assuming the previous regular use of a weak opioid, patients should commence on 200 mcg q8h with the advice that 'If it is not more effective than your previous tablets take a further 200 mcg after one hour, and 400 mcg q8h after that'.

When changing to morphine, multiply the total daily dose of buprenorphine by 60. If the pain was previously poorly relieved, multiply by 100.

Adverse effects, e.g. nausea, vomiting, constipation, drowsiness, need to be monitored as with morphine.

Continuous subcutaneous infusions

When oral administration is no longer feasible, continuous SC infusion of morphine sulphate, diamorphine hydrochloride or hydromorphone obviates the need for injections every four hours (Table 3.9).

Table 3.9: Drugs given by SC infusion

Commonly used	Occasionally used	Not suitable
Diamorphine	Diclofenac[b]	Prochlorperazine[d]
Morphine	Ketorolac[b]	Diazepam[d]
Hydromorphone	Dexamethasone	
Metoclopramide	Methotrimeprazine	
Cyclizine[a]	Chlorpromazine[a]	
Haloperidol	Phenobarbitone[c]	
Hyoscine butylbromide		
Hyoscine hydrobromide		
Midazolam		

a   tends to cause local SC inflammation
b   immiscible with other drugs except diamorphine in saline
c   immiscible with other drugs except diamorphine and hyoscine
d   too irritant for SC use.

Indications for use

- intractable vomiting
- severe dysphagia
- patient too weak to swallow oral drugs
- poor alimentary absorption (*rare*).

Advantages

- constant analgesia (no peaks or troughs)
- usually reloaded once in 24 hours

- comfort and confidence (no repeated injections)
- does not limit mobility
- permits better control of nausea and vomiting.

Choice of infusion sites

- upper chest (intercostal plane)
- upper arm (outer aspect)
- abdomen
- thighs.

If the infusion causes painful local inflammation, consider

- changing needle site prophylactically, e.g. daily
- reducing quantity of the irritant drug
- changing to an alternative drug, e.g. cyclizine to hyoscine
- giving irritant drug IM or PR.

Neuropathic pain

Neuropathic pain is pain associated with neuropathy, i.e. nerve compression and nerve injury (somatic, visceral, sympathetic) or CNS lesions. Pain in an area of abnormal or absent sensation is always neuropathic.

Pathogenesis

There are many causes of neuropathic pain in cancer (Table 3.10). Such pain stems from three different mechanisms.

Table 3.10:   Neuropathic pain in cancer patients

Caused by cancer	Related to cancer and/or debility
Nerve compression/infiltration	Postherpetic neuralgia
Plexopathy	
Spinal cord compression	
Thalamic tumour	
Caused by treatment	Concurrent
Postoperative incisional pain	Diabetic neuropathy
Phantom limb pain	Poststroke pain
Chemotherapy (peripheral neuropathy)	
Radiation (brachial plexopathy)	

Nerve compression

For example nerve root compression caused by a collapsed vertebra.

Nerve injury

For example brachial and lumbosacral plexus infiltration by cancer. This may evolve from earlier nerve compression.

Nerve injury causes pain as a result of

- neuronal hyperexcitability:
     spontaneous activity
     mechanical sensitivity
     alpha-adrenergic sensitivity

- a cascade of neurochemical and physiological changes in the CNS, particularly in the dorsal horn of the spinal cord.

Nerve injury does *not* always lead to pain, e.g. postherpetic neuralgia is rare in young people. Further, with identical lesions, only a minority develops pain. A genetic factor has been postulated.

Sympathetically mediated pain

This is a rare form of neuropathic pain, related to sympathetic nerve trauma at operation or 'irritation' by a tumour. It is similar to somatic nerve injury pain but has an arterial distribution instead of a neuro-dermatomal one. It differs also in its response to treatment.

Clinical characteristics

Distribution

- neurodermatomal, if peripheral lesion.

Quality

- superficial burning/stinging pain, particularly if peripheral lesion; +/– spontaneous stabbing/shooting pain. There may also be a deep aching component.

Concomitants

- often receiving morphine with little effect; often exhausted because of insomnia
- allodynia (light touch exacerbates pain); unable to bear clothing against affected area
- sensory deficits, e.g. numbness
- sometimes there is a sympathetic component manifesting as autonomic instability, i.e. cutaneous vasodilation, increased skin temperature, changes in sweating pattern.

Management

Explanation

Nerve compression pain

- needs cortisone as well as painkillers.

Nerve injury pain

- often does not respond well to painkillers such as aspirin and morphine
- need to start a different type of painkiller
- first step is to get a good night's sleep.

Drugs of choice

Nerve compression pain
A combination of morphine and a corticosteroid, e.g. dexamethasone 4–8 mg daily, is often effective (Figure 3.3).

Nerve injury pain
Often relatively resistant to morphine and corticosteroids. When this is so, it is necessary to use one or more 'secondary analgesics', i.e. drugs not marketed primarily as analgesics but of proven value in relieving nerve injury (Figure 3.4).

- as a general rule, use a tricyclic antidepressant for superficial burning pain and allodynia
- as a general rule, use an anticonvulsant for spontaneous stabbing/shooting pain
- if both types of pain are present, use *either* an antidepressant *or* an anticonvulsant before proceeding to both (step 2)
- some centres use a class 1 cardiac anti-arrhythmic, e.g. flecainide or mexiletine – styled step 3 here – as the drug of choice for nerve

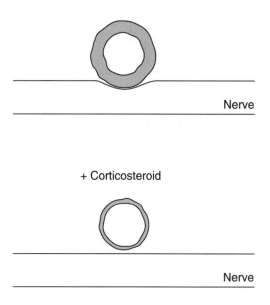

Figure 3.3: Possible mechanism of action of corticosteroids in relief of nerve compression pain. Total tumour mass = neoplasm + surrounding inflammation. General anti-inflammatory effect of corticosteroid reduces total tumour mass resulting in reduction of pain.

Figure 3.4: An analgesic ladder for nerve injury pain.

injury pain, i.e. it is used as step 1. These are chemically related to local anaesthetics

- other centres move straight from step 2 to step 4 (spinal analgesia)
- spinal analgesia includes both epidural and intrathecal routes
- nerve injury pain is more responsive to spinal morphine than morphine by conventional routes. (Spinal analgesia is also used occasionally in patients with nociceptive pain who experience intolerable adverse effects with PO or SC morphine)
- epidural morphine + bupivacaine +/− clonidine by continuous infusion is one commonly used form of spinal analgesia in cancer patients
- in patients who decline spinal analgesia, ketamine (a dissociative anaesthetic and N-methyl D-aspartate/NMDA receptor blocker) can be given in subanaesthetic doses by SC infusion
- some patients benefit from *Transcutaneous Electrical Nerve Stimulation* (TENS)
- the putative mechanisms of various secondary analgesics are shown in Figure 3.5.

Sympathetically mediated pain
Responds to sympathetic nerve blocks (stellate ganglion or lumbar sympathetic chain); does not respond to secondary analgesics.

Therapeutic guidelines

Tricyclic antidepressant e.g. amitriptyline 25–75 mg nocte
Rate of increase in dose depends on pain intensity and extent of supervision. Onset of relief unusual before day four or five and uncommon with 25 mg. It is unusual to need more than 50–75 mg in cancer related neuropathic pain. Maximum dose is determined by the degree of relief and by adverse effects. Adverse effects are a common limiting factor. Mechanism of analgesic action is principally by facilitation of descending inhibitory pathways (Figures 3.5 and 3.6).

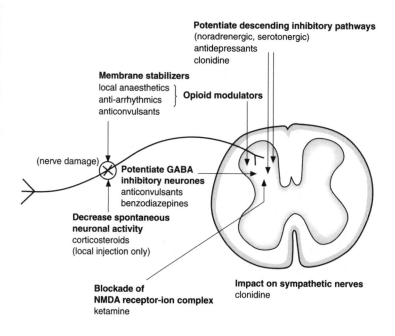

Figure 3.5: Impact of secondary analgesics on peripheral nerves and the dorsal horn of the spinal cord.

Anticonvulsant e.g. sodium valproate 200–1000 mg nocte or carbamazepine
The dose of carbamazepine should be built up slowly from 100 mg b.d. to minimize adverse effects (drowsiness, ataxia, diplopia). Increments should be restricted to 200 mg/week.

- dextropropoxyphene (in co-proxamol) enhances the action of carbamazepine

- some selective serotonin re-uptake inhibitors (SSRIs) increase plasma carbamazepine and valproic acid concentrations; paroxetine does not

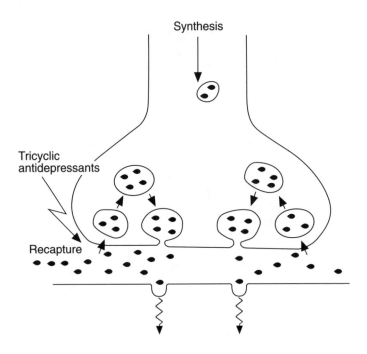

Figure 3.6:   Mono-amine neurotransmission at a neuronal synapse (noradrenaline or serotonin/5-hydroxytryptamine). Tricyclics potentiate two descending inhibitory pathways from the brain (one noradrenergic, the other serotonergic) by blocking presynaptic re-uptake. They also potentiate opioid analgesia by a serotonergic mechanism in the brain stem.

- tricyclic antidepressant metabolism accelerated by carbamazepine
- sodium valproate inhibits the metabolism of tricyclics.

Anti-arrhythmic e.g. flecainide 50–150 mg b.d. or mexiletine 50–300 mg t.d.s.
Major disadvantage is the negative inotropic effect on the heart. *Should not be given to patients with evidence of cardiac failure.* Toxicity includes confusion, paraesthesiae, multifocal myoclonus, fitting and coma. Use smaller doses in renal failure. Risk of pro-arrhythmic effect if used with a tricyclic.

Expectations

About 75% of patients respond well to step 1–3 drugs; the rest require spinal analgesia or other measures to obtain adequate relief.

Response is not an 'all or none' phenomenon. The crucial first step in many cases is to help the patient obtain a good night's sleep with step 1 or 2 drugs. The second is to reduce pain intensity and allodynia to a bearable level during the day. Initially, benefit may be for only part of each day. Adverse effects tend to be the limiting therapeutic factor.

The patient should be warned that results usually take a week or more to become apparent, although improvement in sleep should occur immediately.

Useful definitions

Pharmacological terms	
Receptor affinity ('potency')	A term used to describe the power of attraction between the drug and the drug receptor. Affinity determines the dose of drug required to produce a certain level of biological effect.
Intrinsic activity ('efficacy')	The degree to which the drug is able to stimulate a receptor and thereby produce a biological effect. Intrinsic activity is a basic property of all drugs which act through receptors.
Full agonist	A drug which when bound to the receptor stimulates the receptor to the maximum level, e.g. morphine. By definition the intrinsic activity of a full agonist is unity.
Pure antagonist	A drug which when bound to the receptor fails completely to produce any stimulation of that receptor, e.g. naloxone. By definition the intrinsic activity of a pure antagonist is zero.
Partial agonist	A drug which when bound to the receptor stimulates the receptor to a level below the maximum level, e.g. buprenorphine (partial mu agonist). By definition the intrinsic activity of a partial agonist lies between zero and unity.

continued

Mixed agonist -antagonist	A drug which acts simultaneously on different types of receptor, with the potential for agonist action on one or more types and antagonist action on one or more types, e.g. pentazocine (partial mu agonist + kappa agonist + weak delta antagonist).
Ligand	A substance which binds to a receptor. (The use of this term circumvents the need to say whether the substance is an agonist or an antagonist.)

Pain terms (IASP, 1994)

Allodynia	Pain caused by a stimulus which does not normally provoke pain.
Anaesthesia dolorosa	Pain in an area which is numb.
Analgesia	Absence of pain in response to stimulation which would normally be painful.
Causalgia	A syndrome of sustained burning pain, allodynia, and hyperpathia after a traumatic nerve lesion, often combined with vasomotor and sudomotor dysfunction and later trophic changes.
Central pain	Pain associated with a lesion of the CNS.
Dysaesthesia	An unpleasant abnormal sensation, whether spontaneous or evoked.

continued

Hyperaesthesia	Increased sensitivity to stimulation.
Hyperalgesia	An increased response to a stimulus which is normally painful.
Hyperpathia	A painful syndrome characterized by increased reaction to a stimulus, especially a repetitive stimulus, *as well as an increased threshold*. (This latter feature results in a delayed onset. It tends to be poorly localized and outlasts the stimulus.)
Neuralgia	Pain in the distribution of a nerve.
Neuropathy	A disturbance of function or a pathological change in a nerve.
Nociceptor	A receptor preferentially sensitive to a noxious stimulus or to a stimulus which would become noxious if prolonged.
Noxious stimulus	A noxious stimulus is one which is damaging to normal tissues.
Pain	An unpleasant sensory and emotional experience associated with actual or potential tissue damage or described in terms of such damage.
Pain threshold	The least experience of pain which a subject can recognize.
Pain tolerance level	The greatest level of pain which a subject is prepared to tolerate.

PART FOUR

Symptom Management II

Alimentary symptoms
Respiratory symptoms
Urinary symptoms · Other symptoms
Secondary mental disorders
Drug profiles

Alimentary symptoms

Dyspepsia

Definition

Retrosternal, epigastric, or more general abdominal discomfort following a meal. Synonyms include acid indigestion and upset stomach.

Pathogenesis

There are many causes of dyspepsia (Table 4.1). From a therapeutic perspective dyspepsia in advanced cancer can be divided into three categories

- gassy
- acid
- dysmotility.

It is important to decide which type of dyspepsia a patient is suffering from because the treatment is dependent on the cause. Careful history taking will usually indicate which type is predominant. Some patients with dysmotility dyspepsia also have symptoms or a history of irritable bowel syndrome.

Table 4.1:   Causes of dyspepsia in advanced cancer

Caused by cancer	*Related to cancer and/or debility*
Gastric cancer	Oesophageal candidiasis
Squashed stomach syndrome	Minimal food and fluid intake
Gastroparesis (autonomic neuropathy)	Anxiety → aerophagia
Caused by treatment	*Concurrent*

Postsurgical
  small stomach syndrome
  reflux oesophagitis
	Organic dyspepsia
	  peptic ulcer
	  reflux oesophagitis
	  cholelithiasis
	  renal failure

Irradiation
  lumbar spine
  epigastrium
	Non-ulcer dyspepsia

Drugs
  physical irritant (→ gastritis)
    iron
    metronidazole
    tranexamic acid
  acid stimulant (→ gastritis)
    NSAIDs
    corticosteroids
  delayed gastric emptying
    anticholinergics
    opioids
    cisplatin	

Treatment

Gassy dyspepsia
Prescribe an antiflatulent, e.g. activated dimethicone. This is available on its own but may conveniently be given in the form of Asilone, a proprietary antacid (*see* p.150). Depending on a patient's individual needs, this can be given 'as needed', q.d.s., or both.

Acid dyspepsia
Prescribe an antacid, an H_2 receptor blocker (e.g. cimetidine, ranitidine) or a proton pump inhibitor (omeprazole) according to the patient's individual circumstances.

In patients taking a NSAID, misoprostol (a prostaglandin analogue) should be used for dyspepsia, 200 mcg q.d.s. or 400 mcg b.d. If used prophylactically to prevent NSAID gastropathy in patients with a history of peptic ulceration, 200 mcg b.d. is normally adequate.

Dysmotility dyspepsia
This is not helped by antacids, H_2 receptor blockers or omeprazole. Treatment is with a prokinetic drug, i.e. metoclopramide, domperidone, cisapride. These normalize the disordered gastric motility.

Squashed stomach syndrome

Definition

Dyspeptic symptoms associated with the inability of the stomach to distend normally because of hepatomegaly (Table 4.2). Similar symptoms may be seen with cancer of the stomach, linitis plastica, or postgastrectomy ('small stomach syndrome').

Table 4.2:   Symptoms of squashed stomach syndrome

Early satiety	Hiccup
Epigastric fullness	Nausea
Epigastric discomfort/pain	Vomiting (particularly post-prandial)
Flatulence	
	Heartburn

Treatment

- explanation
- dietary advice, e.g. 'small and often', separate main food and main fluid intake
- antiflatulent, i.e. activated dimethicone (as in Asilone) with meals and bedtime
- prokinetic drug, e.g. metoclopramide, with meals and bedtime.

Nausea and vomiting

There are many potential causes of nausea and vomiting in advanced cancer (Figure 4.1). It is important to identify the most likely cause(s) in each patient because the treatment is dependent on the cause.

On the basis of putative sites of action (Table 4.3), it is possible to derive anti-emetic drugs of choice for different situations (Table 4.4).

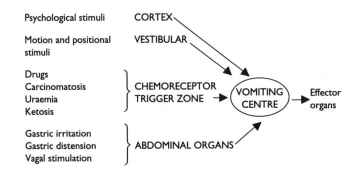

Figure 4.1: Causes of vomiting. The chemoreceptor trigger zone and the vomiting centre are located in the floor of the fourth ventricle.

Table 4.3: Anti-emetic classification

Putative site of action	Class	Example
Vomiting centre	Anticholinergic	Hyoscine hydrobromide
	Antihistamine	Cyclizine Dimenhydrinate
Chemoreceptor trigger zone	Dopamine (D_2) antagonist	Haloperidol, Prochlorperazine Metoclopramide Domperidone
Upper gastrointestinal tract	$5HT_4$ agonist	Metoclopramide Cisapride
	Dopamine (D_2) antagonist	Metoclopramide Domperidone
Upper gastrointestinal tract	$5HT_3$ antagonist	Ondansetron Granisetron
Cerebral cortex	Benzodiazepine Cannabinoid	Lorazepam Nabilone
Unknown	Corticosteroid	Dexamethasone

Table 4.4: Anti-emetics in advanced cancer

Cause of nausea/vomiting	Anti-emetic of choice	Comment
Drug induced	Haloperidol 1.5–3 mg nocte or Prochlorperazine 5–10 mg q8h	Adverse effects unusual at lower doses
Radiotherapy		
Chemotherapy		
Metabolic uraemia hypercalcaemia	Haloperidol 5–20 mg/day	May cause dry mouth and mild drowsiness; extrapyramidal effects sometimes occur
Raised intracranial pressure	Cyclizine or dimenhydrinate 50–100 mg t.d.s.	Anticholinergic effects; may cause drowsiness
Bowel obstruction	Cyclizine or dimenhydrinate 50–100 mg t.d.s. or Hyoscine butylbromide 60–120 mg SC/24 h or Octreotide 300–600 mcg SC/24 h	Anticholinergic effects; may cause drowsiness Anticholinergic effects

continued

Table 4.4: *Continued*

Cause of nausea/vomiting	Anti-emetic of choice	Comment
Oesophageal reflux	Metoclopramide 10–20 mg t.d.s.–q4h *or* Domperidone 10–20 mg t.d.s.–q4h *or*	Do not cause anticholinergic effects; extrapyramidal effects seen only with metoclopramide
Delayed gastric emptying	Cisapride 20 mg b.d.–t.d.s.	
Gastric irritation by drug	Treat gastritis Modify medication	Sometimes seen with NSAIDs and corticosteroids

Constipation

Constipation (difficult defaecation) is common in advanced cancer. Diminished food and fibre intake, lack of exercise and drugs which constipate all contribute to its development. As with nausea and vomiting, it is necessary to be aware of the different classes of laxatives (Table 4.5) and to know what are the laxatives of choice in different circumstances.

Table 4.5:   Classification of laxatives

Bulk forming drugs	Osmotic laxatives
Ispaghula husk (Fybogel, Regulan)	Lactulose syrup
Methylcellulose	Magnesium hydroxide suspension (Milk of magnesia)
Sterculia (Normacol)	Magnesium sulphate (Epsom salts)
Faecal softeners	
Surface wetting agents docusate sodium poloxamer	Liquid paraffin and magnesium hydroxide oral emulsion BP
	Stimulant laxatives (colonic)
Lubricants liquid paraffin/mineral oil	Senna
	Danthron
	Bisacodyl
	Sodium picosulphate

Patients not on constipating drugs may be satisfactorily treated with senna or bisacodyl tablets. Those receiving morphine often do well with co-danthrusate or strong co-danthramer, i.e. a combination of a stimulant laxative (danthron) and a softener.

Management of opioid induced constipation

- ask patient about usual bowel habit and use of laxatives
- do rectal examination if suspect faecal impaction or if diarrhoea/ faecal incontinence (to exclude impaction with overflow)
- record bowel motions each day in 'Bowel Book'
- encourage fluids generally, fruit juice, fruit and bran
- prescribe prophylactically, co-danthrusate 1 capsule nocte
- if already constipated, co-danthrusate 2 capsules nocte
- adjust every few days according to results, up to 2 capsules q.d.s
- if necessary 'uncork' with the help of bisacodyl 10 mg suppository + glycerine suppository
- if suppositories are ineffective, administer a high phosphate enema
- if the maximum dose of co-danthrusate is ineffective, reduce by half and add an osmotic laxative, e.g. lactulose syrup 30 ml b.d.
- if co-danthrusate causes abdominal cramps divide daily dose or change to an osmotic laxative, e.g. lactulose syrup 20–40 ml daily–t.d.s.
- lactulose may be preferable to co-danthrusate in patients with a history of irritable bowel syndrome or of colic with other colonic stimulants, e.g. senna
- sometimes it is appropriate to optimize a patient's existing bowel regimen, rather than change automatically to co-danthrusate
- if patient prefers a liquid preparation, use strong co-danthramer suspension.

Bowel obstruction

The focus here is on patients in whom available oncological therapies for tumour control have been exhausted.

Causes

- the cancer itself
- past treatment, e.g. adhesions, postradiation, ischaemic fibrosis
- associated with debility, e.g. constipation
- an unrelated benign condition, e.g. strangulated hernia
- a combination of factors.

In consequence, bowel obstruction may be

- mechanical *or* functional *or* both
- high *or* low *or* both
- single *or* multiple sites
- partial *or* complete
- transient *or* persistent.

Clinical features

Continuous abdominal pain caused by the underlying cancer is almost always present. Vomiting occurs in about 80% and intestinal colic in about the same proportion. Distension is variable and bowel habit ranges from absolute constipation to diarrhoea. Bowel sounds vary considerably – from absent in an ileus to hyperactive (borborygmi). Tinkling bowel sounds are not common in this group of patients.

Surgical management

Surgical intervention is *contra-indicated* if there is

- intra-abdominal carcinomatosis as evidenced by diffuse intra-abdominal tumours
- massive ascites which re-accumulates rapidly after paracentesis.[32]

Surgical intervention should be considered if the following criteria are fulfilled

- the patient's general condition is good, i.e. does not have widely disseminated disease and has been independent and active
- previous laparotomy findings do not preclude the prospect of successful intervention
- an easily reversible cause seems likely, e.g. postoperative adhesions or a single discrete neoplastic obstruction
- the patient is willing to undergo surgery.

Medical management

In patients in whom an operative approach is contra-indicated, it is generally possible to relieve symptoms adequately with drugs. A nasogastric tube and IV fluids are rarely necessary.

Eliminate pain and colic

- administer diamorphine by continuous SC infusion using a portable syringe driver for constant background pain
- if the patient is experiencing colic:
  do not use a prokinetic drug
  discontinue bulk forming osmotic and stimulant laxatives
- if colic persists despite SC diamorphine, prescribe SC hyoscine butylbromide (Buscopan) 60–120 mg/24 h as well.

Eliminate nausea and reduce vomiting to once or twice a day
The choice of anti-emetic depends on whether the patient is experiencing colic. If yes, hyoscine butylbromide will have been started already. If no, the following sequence can be followed

- if passing flatus, a *trial* of SC metoclopramide 60–160 mg/24 h helps to determine whether the obstruction is more functional than mechanical

- if not helpful, prescribe SC cyclizine 100–150 mg/24 h

- if cyclizine fails, hyoscine butylbromide should be tried because of its antisecretory properties

- octreotide 300–600 mcg/24 h may be used instead. This is a somatostatin analogue with similar intestinal effects to hyoscine butylbromide but no anticholinergic effects; it is expensive

- if there is persistent nausea (often caused by toxic factors), add haloperidol 5–10 mg/24 h

- a venting gastrostomy is only occasionally needed

- some centres recommend SC methotrimeprazine 50–150 mg/24 h when all else fails; half the patients experience sedation.

Relieve associated constipation
Enemas: high phosphate enema. Repeat once or twice in case concurrent constipation is playing a significant causal role.

Laxatives: prescribe docusate tablets 100–200 mg b.d. If small bowel only affected, consider colonic stimulant laxative.

General
Inoperable patients managed by drug therapy should be encouraged to drink and eat small amounts of their favourite beverages and food. Some patients find that they can manage food best in the morning.

The use of anticholinergic drugs and diminished fluid intake often result in a dry mouth and thirst. These symptoms are usually relieved by conscientious mouth care. A few ml of fluid every 30–40 min, possibly administered as a small ice cube, often brings relief. IV hydration is rarely needed.

Ascites

Ascites can cause several symptoms of differing intensity (Table 4.6).

Table 4.6: Clinical features of ascites

Abdominal distension	Acid reflux
Abdominal discomfort/pain	Nausea and vomiting
Inability to sit upright	Leg oedema
Squashed stomach syndrome	Dyspnoea

Pathogenesis

- usually associated with peritoneal metastases
- subphrenic lymphatics become blocked by tumour infiltration
- increased peritoneal permeability
- hyperaldosteronism, possibly secondary to reduced extracellular blood volume, causes sodium retention and further feeds the ascitic process
- liver metastases leading to hypo-albuminaemia and, sometimes, portal hypertension.

Treatment options

Chemotherapy (systemic or intraperitoneal)
Diuretics (Table 4.7)

Table 4.7:   Diuretic treatment of malignant ascites

	Spironolactone	Loop diuretic	
		Bumetanide or Frusemide	
Day 1	100–200 mg o.d.	–	–
Day 7	200–300 mg o.d.	1 mg	40 mg
Day 14	200 mg b.d.	2 mg	80 mg

The dose of the loop diuretic should be reduced once a satisfactory result is achieved.

Failure with diuretic therapy usually relates to

- gastric intolerance (spironolactone)
- therapeutic impatience
- too small a dose of spironolactone
- failure to use concomitant loop diuretic in resistant cases.

Paracentesis
For a distressed patient with a tense painful abdomen. Remove as much fluid as possible using an IV cannula. Repeat if diuretics do not prevent re-accumulation.

Peritoneovenous shunt
This is an option in a patient who is relatively well but cannot tolerate diuretic therapy. It is not often necessary.

Respiratory symptoms

Dyspnoea

All advanced cancer 50%; lung cancer 70%. Incidence increases in the weeks immediately before death.

Relevant pathophysiology

Various respiratory drives predispose to dyspnoea (Table 4.8).

Table 4.8: Respiratory drives

Wakefulness	Lung deflation
Anxiety, fear	Acidosis
Anger, rage	Hypercapnia
Pyrexia	Hypoxia
Lung distortion	

Respiratory panic attacks cause acute exacerbations usually on exertion, e.g. going upstairs:

dyspnoea + lack of understanding + fear → increased anxiety → increased respiratory rate → increased dyspnoea etc.

Dyspnoea is usually associated with *tachypnoea*. If the resting respiratory rate is 30–35 min, activity or additional anxiety may increase this to 50–60 min.

Dyspnoea is often caused by multiple factors (Table 4.9). A dyspnoeic patient is often an anxious patient, particularly if dyspnoeic at rest.

Table 4.9:   Causes of dyspnoea in advanced cancer

Caused by cancer	Related to cancer and/or debility
Effusion(s)	Anaemia
Obstruction of a main bronchus	Atelectasis
Replacement of lung by cancer	Pulmonary embolism
Lymphangitis	Pneumonia
Mediastinal obstruction	Empyema
Pericardial effusion	Weakness
Massive ascites	
Abdominal distension	*Concurrent*
Cachexia	
	Chronic obstructive pulmonary disease (COPD)
Caused by cancer treatment	Asthma
	Heart failure
Pneumonectomy	Acidosis
Radiation-induced fibrosis	
Chemotherapy	
bleomycin	
adriamycin	

Treatment options

Explanation

Respond to or anticipate patient's questions, e.g. 'Will I choke to death?', 'Will I suffocate?', 'Will I stop breathing if I go to sleep?' Emphasize, 'Becoming breathless in itself is not dangerous'.

Respiratory panic

- prophylactic education about and practice in breathing control

- a calming presence +/– lorazepam 0.5–1 mg SL (for short term relief) or diazepam 5–10 mg PO nocte (for long term relief).

Treat concurrent reversible causes

- bronchospasm   → bronchodilator
- cardiac failure   → diuretic, ACE inhibitor
- infection   → antibiotic (?)
- anaemia (Hb < 10 g/dl)   → transfusion (?).

Modification of pathological process

- fever   → antipyretic
- bronchial obstruction   → corticosteroid
                                  → radiation therapy
                                       external beam
                                       endobronchial
                                  → LASER therapy
                                  → bronchial stent

- chemotherapy
- pleural effusion   → thoracic paracentesis
                                  → pleurodesis

- gross ascites   → abdominal paracentesis.

Nondrug measures

- a calming presence
- cool draught
- breathing exercises
- relaxation therapy.

Modify way of life

- sit to wash/shave
- help with housework

- bed downstairs

- bed rest.

Drugs for dyspnoea

- morphine; the aim is to ease the sensation of dyspnoea:
  if on morphine for pain, consider increasing the dose by 50%
  if not on oral morphine, 5 mg q4h is a good starting dose
  can be given via *nebulizer* 10–40 mg up to q3h (only 5% systemic bio-availability)

- diazepam if the patient is very anxious:
  5–10 mg stat and 5–20 mg nocte
  in the very elderly, 2–5 mg
  reduce dose after several days if drowsy

- oxygen 4 l/min via nasal cannulae if dyspnoeic at rest.

Special situations

Acute tracheal compression/massive haemorrhage into trachea
This is a very rare palliative care emergency

- IV diazepam/midazolam until patient unconscious (5–20 mg)

- PR diazepam or IM midazolam 20 mg, if IV administration not possible

- continuous company.

Noisy tachypnoea in the moribund
Although the patient is not aware, the family and other patients become distressed. Consider slowing the respiratory rate down to 10–15/min with IV diamorphine/morphine. It may be necessary to give double or treble the previously satisfactory analgesic dose to contain this form of tachypnoea. If there is associated heaving of the shoulders and chest, midazolam should be given as well, e.g. 10 mg SC stat and hourly as needed.

Cough

Causes

These include

- intrathoracic cancer
- chest infection
- chronic bronchitis
- cigarettes.

Types of cough

- wet cough and patient able to cough effectively
- wet cough but patient too weak to cough effectively
- dry cough, i.e. not productive of sputum.

Treatment options

Treat concurrent reversible causes

- postnasal drip   ⟶   antihistamine, beclomethasone nasal spray
- bronchospasm   ⟶   bronchodilator
- heart failure   ⟶   diuretic, ACE inhibitor
- infection   ⟶   antibiotic (?)
- cigarettes   ⟶   stop smoking.

It takes two to four weeks to obtain any significant benefit after stopping smoking. Will the patient live as long as this?

Modification of pathological process

- corticosteroids
- radiation therapy
- chemotherapy.

Nondrug measures

- advise how to cough effectively; it is impossible to cough effectively lying on your back
- postural drainage
- physiotherapy.

Mucolytics/expectorants

- saline 2–5% in nebulizer
- chemical inhalations:
  compound benzoin tincture (Friar's balsam)
  carbol
  menthol and eucalyptus
- 'irritant' mucolytics:
  guaiphenesin
  ipecacuanha
  potassium iodide
- chemical mucolytics:
  acetylcysteine
  carbocysteine.

Antitussives

- simple linctus
- codeine linctus
- strong opioid, e.g. morphine, methadone.

Hiccup

Definition

A pathological respiratory reflex characterized by spasm of the diaphragm, resulting in sudden inspiration and associated with closure of the vocal cords.

Causes

There are innumerable potential causes of hiccup. In advanced cancer, the following account for most cases

- gastric distension
- diaphragmatic irritation
- phrenic nerve irritation
- toxicity:
  uraemia
  infection
- CNS tumour.

Of these, gastric distension probably accounts for 95% of cases.

Treatment options for hiccups

Pharyngeal stimulation (triggers a 'gating' mechanism)

- drinking from 'wrong' side of a cup
- granulated sugar (two heaped teaspoons) rapidly ingested
- liqueur (two glasses) rapidly ingested
- cold key down back of neck (acts via hyperextension of neck)
- pulling tongue out of mouth forcibly.

Massage of the junction between hard and soft palate with a cotton bob is also an effective gating mechanism.

Reduce gastric distension

- peppermint water facilitates belching by relaxing lower oesophageal sphincter (an old-fashioned remedy)
- antiflatulent, e.g. Asilone 10 ml
- metoclopramide 10 mg (tightens lower oesophageal sphincter and hastens gastric emptying).

Peppermint water and metoclopramide should not be used concurrently.

Elevation of pCO_2
This inhibits processing of the hiccup reflex in the brain stem

- rebreathing from a paper bag
- breath holding.

Muscle relaxant

- baclofen 10 mg PO
- nifedipine 10 mg PO
- midazolam 5–10 mg IV.

Central suppression of hiccup reflex

- haloperidol 5 mg PO or IV if no response
- chlorpromazine 10–25 mg PO or IV if no response.

The IV route is rarely necessary.

Maintenance treatment

Gastric distension

- antiflatulent, e.g. Asilone 10 ml qds and/or
- metoclopramide 10 mg q.d.s.

Diaphragmatic irritation or other cause

- baclofen 5–10 mg b.d.–20 mg q8h *or*
- nifedipine 10–20 mg q8h *or*
- haloperidol 5–10 mg nocte *or*
- midazolam 10–60 mg/24 h by infusion.

Urinary symptoms

Useful definitions

Frequency	Passage of urine seven or more times during the day and twice or more at night.
Urgency	A strong and sudden desire to void.
Urge incontinence	The involuntary loss of urine associated with a strong desire to void.
Detrusor instability	Detrusor contracts uninhibitedly and causes:

diurnal frequency ⎫
nocturnal frequency ⎬ increasing severity
urgency ⎪
urge incontinence ⎭ ↓
(Detrusor instability is the second most common cause of urinary incontinence in women.)

continued

Stress incontinence	The involuntary loss of urine associated with coughing, sneezing, laughing and lifting.
Genuine stress incontinence (Urethral sphincter incompetence)	The involuntary loss of urine when the intravesical pressure exceeds maximum urethral pressure in the *absence of detrusor activity*. The fault always lies in the sphincter mechanisms of the bladder, and is associated with multiparity, postmenopause and posthysterectomy.
	One or more of the following features will be present:
	descent of urethrovesical junction outside intra-abdominal zone of pressure decrease in urethral pressure due to loss of urethral wall elasticity and contractility short functional length of the urethra. (Urethral sphincter incompetence is the most common cause of urinary incontinence in women.)

Urinary bladder innervation

'You pee with your parasympathetics.
You stop with your sympathetics.'

The sphincter relaxes when the detrusor (bladder muscle) contracts, and vice versa (Table 4.10). Thus, anticholinergic (antimuscarinic) drugs not only cause contraction of the bladder neck sphincter but also relax the detrusor.

Table 4.10:   Autonomic innervation of urinary bladder

		Effect on	
Innervation	Mediator	Sphincter	Vault
Sympathetic (T10–12, L1)	Noradrenaline	Contracts (alpha)	Relaxes (beta)
Parasympathetic (S2–4)	Acetylcholine	Relaxes	Contracts

Detrusor sensitivity is

- increased by prostaglandins
- decreased by cyclo-oxygenase inhibitors (NSAIDs).

The external sphincter (urethral) is an additional voluntary mechanism innervated by the pudendal nerve (S2–4).

The urethra, derived embryologically from the urogenital sinus, is sensitive in the female to oestrogen and progesterone. Post-menopausal urge incontinence and frequency is sometimes helped by the prescription of an oestrogen, either topically or orally. Oestrogens do not improve stress incontinence.

Morphine and other opioids have several effects on bladder function (Table 4.11). These are usually asymptomatic. Occasionally hesitancy will develop and/or retention precipitated.

Causes

The most common urinary symptoms in advanced cancer are

- frequency and urgency
- incontinence

Table 4.11:   Morphine and the urinary tract

Bladder sensation decreased
Sphincter tone *increased*
Detrusor tone *increased*
Ureteric tone and amplitude of contractions increased

- hesitancy and retention
- bladder spasms.

Causes to be considered are listed in Tables 4.12–4.15. As in other areas of symptom management, careful evaluation is fundamental. Rectal examination to exclude faecal impaction may be necessary in debilitated/moribund patients, particularly if there is associated delirium.

Treatment

Treatment depends on the cause and commonly comprises both nondrug and drug approaches. The detection and treatment of urinary infection is obviously important if causing dysuria, urgency and frequency. 'Bladder drill' (e.g. voiding every two hours by the clock) may be helpful in someone with urge incontinence.

Drugs of choice

Urgency
Consider

- oxybutynin 2.5–5 mg b.d.–q.d.s. *or*
- amitriptyline 25–50 mg nocte *or*
- propantheline 15 mg b.d.–t.d.s.

Treatment may be limited by anticholinergic effects.

Table 4.12:   Causes of urgency and incontinence

Caused by cancer	*Related to cancer and/or debility*
Pain	Infective cystitis
Hypercalcaemia (causes polyuria)	*Concurrent*
Intravesical } mechanical Extravesical } irritation	Idiopathic detrusor instability

	Central neurological disease
	    poststroke
	    multiple sclerosis
	    dementia

Bladder spasms	
Sacral plexopathy	
	Uraemia } cause Diabetes mellitus } polyuria Diabetes insipidus }
Caused by treatment	
Radiation cystitis	
Cyclophosphamide cystitis	

Drugs
    diuretics
    (opioids)	

Hesitancy
Consider

- indoramin 20 mg nocte–b.d., a selective alpha-1 adrenoceptor antagonist (maximum daily dose 100 mg)
- bethanechol 10–30 mg b.d.–q.d.s., a cholinergic drug.

Table 4.13:   Causes of hesitancy and retention

Caused by cancer	*Related to cancer and/or debility*
Malignant enlargement of prostate	Loaded rectum
	Inability to stand to void
Infiltration of bladder neck	Generalized weakness
Presacral plexopathy	*Concurrent*
Spinal cord compression	Benign enlargement of prostate
Caused by treatment	
Anticholinergic drugs (*see* p.157)	
Morphine (occasionally)	
Spinal analgesia (particularly with bupivacaine)	
Intrathecal nerve block	

Table 4.14:   Causes of bladder spasms

Caused by cancer	*Related to cancer and/or debility*
Intravesical } irritation Extravesical }	Anxiety
	Infective cystitis
Caused by treatment	Indwelling catheter
Radiation fibrosis	mechanical irritation by catheter balloon
	catheter sludging with partial retention

Bladder spasm

- if catheterized, change catheter or reduce volume of balloon
- if urinary infection:
    no catheter – treat with systemic antibiotic
    catheter – treat with bladder washouts and/or urinary antiseptics,
        e.g. hexamine hippurate 1 g b.d.
- anticholinergic drug (as for urgency)
- flavoxate 200–400 mg t.d.s.–q.d.s. (a weak detrusor relaxant) if anticholinergic drugs cause unacceptable adverse effects.

Discoloured urine

There are many causes of discoloured urine (Table 4.15). The patient and family fear that it is evidence of further deterioration. If red, it is assumed to be haematuria.

Table 4.15:   Common causes of discoloured urine

Cause	Colour
Diet	
Rhubarb	Red
Beetroot	Red
Drugs	
Adriamycin	Red
Danthron	Red/green/blue
Phenolphthalein	Pink (alkaline urine)

Other symptoms

Hypercalcaemia

Hypercalcaemia may cause various symptoms, e.g. dry mouth, nausea and vomiting, constipation, frequency (polyuria), lethargy, weakness and/or depression.

Incidence

All malignant disease 10%; squamous cancer of the bronchus, breast cancer, myeloma 20–40%.

Diagnosis is based on a high level of clinical suspicion and confirmed by blood tests, 'correcting' for hypo-albuminaemia.

Stop and think!

It is sometimes appropriate to regard severe symptomatic hypercalcaemia as the terminal event. The following together comprise a set of indications for the urgent correction of hypercalcaemia

- severe symptoms attributable to hypercalcaemia
- first episode or long interval since previous one
- previous good quality of life (in patient's opinion)
- medical judgement that measures will achieve a durable effect (based on the results of previous treatment)
- patient willing to undergo IV therapy and requisite blood tests.

Treatment

IV rehydration with normal saline, e.g. 3 l/24 h, and IV bisphosphonate, e.g. pamidronate 30–45 mg or clodronate 1500 mg by infusion in saline over 2–8 hours

- bisphosphonates act by inhibiting osteoclasts
- maximum effect 5–7 days with pamidronate; 3–5 days with clodronate
- repeat after 4–7 days if initial poor response
- effect usually lasts several weeks with pamidronate; less with clodronate.

Spinal cord compression

Above L1–L2: true cord compression (paraplegia).

Below L1–L2: cauda equina compression (peripheral nerves only affected).

Incidence

An uncommon but potentially devastating phenomenon. Most occur in the thoracic region. Compression occurs at more than one level in 20% of cases. Cancers of the breast and bronchus and lymphoma account for 40% of cases.

Presentation

- pain   > 90%
- weakness   > 75%
- sensory level   > 50%
- sphincter dysfunction > 40%.

The patient may be unaware of sensory loss until examined, particularly if this is confined to sacral or perineal areas.

Pain may relate to

- local bone pain
- root compression pain
- cord compression pain (cuff or garter pain around thighs, knees and/or calves).

Diagnosis

- history and clinical findings
- a plain radiograph shows vertebral metastasis and/or collapse in 80%
- a bone scan does not often yield additional information
- MRI is the investigation of choice
- CT with myelography may be helpful if MRI is not available.

Treatment

- dexamethasone; the dose used varies greatly. One regimen is 12 mg PO stat and then 16–32 mg daily for 1 week; after which it is reduced/stopped over the next 2–3 weeks
- radiation therapy concurrently
- decompressive laminectomy; consider if:
  diagnosis in doubt
  solitary vertebral metastasis
  relapse after maximum radiation given.

If the cord compression is of rapid onset (1–2 days), the most likely cause is infarction of the spinal cord as a consequence of spinal artery thrombosis secondary to compression/distortion by malignant disease. This does not respond to treatment.

Lymphoedema

Definition

Excessive interstitial fluid with a high protein content associated with chronic inflammation and fibrosis.

Lymphoedema can occur in any part of the body, usually a limb with or without adjacent trunk involvement. It is progressive and, if left untreated, becomes a gross and debilitating condition. Acute inflammation (whether infective or not) and trauma cause a rapid increase in swelling.

Causes

Lymphoedema may be

- primary, e.g. congenital, hereditary (Milroy's disease), sporadic
- secondary, e.g. cancer and anticancer treatments, infections, trauma.

In the UK, cancer and anticancer treatment account for most cases of secondary lymphoedema, i.e.

- axillary or groin surgery
- postoperative infection
- radiotherapy
- axillary, groin or intrapelvic recurrence.

Clinical features

- a swollen limb which does not resolve with elevation
- if acute, will pit on pressure; when chronic, less or no pitting
- impaired limb mobility and function
- pain related to tissue swelling and/or shoulder strain. May be concurrent neuropathic pain if there is recurrence in the axilla
- psychological distress because of altered body image, unsightliness and inability to wear short sleeved garments or shoes.

Management

Skin hygiene

- apply cream to skin after gentle washing and drying, e.g. aqueous cream; best done at bedtime
- topical treatment of fungal infection; if persistent, seek advice from a dermatologist
- systemic treatment of bacterial infection, e.g. penicillin V, erythromycin or cephalexin 500 mg q.d.s. Continue for 2 weeks because of stagnant lymph and impaired immunity.

External compression

- initial intensive phase with multilayer short stretch compression bandaging to reshape limb and reduce size; not always necessary (Table 4.16)
- maintenance phase with an 'off the shelf' containment garment.

Table 4.16:   Indications for initial intensive treatment

Grossly swollen limb
Awkwardly shaped limb, i.e. very deep skin folds
Involvement of fingers
Involvement of trunk
Persistent copious lymphorrhoea (lymph leakage)
Severe pain caused by the swelling
Recurrent acute inflammatory episodes

Exercise

- encourage normal use of the limb
- daily exercise of the affected limb
- increasing range of movements
- general increase in physical activity.

Patients must wear compression bandaging or a containment garment during exercise.

The compression enhances the effect of muscle contraction on lymph flow and surface friction stimulates contractions in the superficial lymphatics.

Light massage

Light skin-moving manual trunk massage stimulates skin lymphatics to contract, thereby increasing superficial lymph flow away from the swollen limb.

Other

- a diuretic should be used if the swelling developed or worsened after the prescription of a NSAID or a corticosteroid, or if there is a venous component. Otherwise, do *not* prescribe because it will have no effect on protein-rich oedema

- a pneumatic compression pump is helpful in shifting *venous* oedema. Its use may speed up the rate of initial improvement in patients with combined lymphovenous oedema.

Pruritus

Causes

- dry flaky skin (xerosis)
- wet macerated skin
- concurrent skin disease
- drug reaction
- cholestatic jaundice
- renal failure
- paraneoplastic
- diabetes – usually localized and related to candidiasis
- psychiatric.

Treatment

A dry skin is almost always present in patients with advanced cancer who experience pruritus, even when there is a definite endogenous cause. Measures to correct skin dryness should precede specific measures, or go hand in hand with them.

Pruritus in renal failure is often more difficult to treat. It is associated with an increase in dermal mast cells and divalent ions (magnesium and calcium). In patients with hypercalcaemia associated with secondary hyperparathyroidism, correction of hypercalcaemia leads to the rapid relief of pruritus.

General measures

- discourage scratching; cut nails if necessary; allow gentle rubbing
- discontinue use of soap
- use emulsifying ointment or aqueous cream as a soap substitute, or add Oilatum to bath water
- avoid hot, long baths
- dry skin gently by patting with soft towel
- avoid overheating and sweating.

Topical measures for worst affected areas

- aqueous cream applied to skin after bath and each evening
- clioquinol (Vioform)-hydrocortisone cream if inflamed b.d.–t.d.s.
- crotamiton (Eurax) cream b.d.–t.d.s. has both mild antipruritic and antiscabetic properties. It is rarely necessary.

Drugs
These are of little benefit if used without skin care

- most patients with advanced cancer and pruritus never need an antihistamine if given appropriate skin care
- in obstructive jaundice, an androgen, e.g. stanozolol 5–10 mg daily, eases pruritus in 5–10 days.

Cholestyramine (an anion-exchange resin which binds bile acids) is *not* recommended. Most patients find it unpalatable and it is of no value in obstructive jaundice.

Secondary mental disorders

Definition

Mental disorders which are secondary to organic disease or related to chemical substances (drugs, alcohol) or both. Synonym: organic mental disorders.

Classification

Secondary mental disorders are classified mainly on the basis of their key features (Table 4.17).

Table 4.17:   Secondary mental disorders

Delirium	Hallucinosis
Dementia	Delusional disorder
Amnestic disorder	Personality disorder
Anxiety disorder	Intoxication
Mood disorder	Withdrawal state

All secondary mental disorders may be seen in patients with advanced cancer.

Delirium (synonyms: acute brain syndrome, acute confusional state), dementia (synonym: chronic brain syndrome) and secondary amnestic disorder are all characterized by cognitive impairment. The word 'confusion' is often used of all three conditions. Note that

- sometimes dementia is compounded by delirium
- dementia is not usually associated with somnolence
- some patients with cancer appear to develop dementia rapidly – and this may cause difficulty in diagnosis (Table 4.18).

Patients with cognitive impairment disorders have identifiable cognitive defects if tested formally using, for example, the Mini-Mental State Examination.

Table 4.18:   Comparison of global cognitive impairment disorders

Delirium		Dementia	
Acute		Chronic	
Often remitting and reversible		Usually progressive and irreversible	
Mental clouding (information not taken in)		Brain damage (information not retained)	
	+	Poor concentration	+
	+	Impaired short term memory	+
	+	Disorientation	+
	+	Living in the past	+
	+	Misinterpretations	+
	++	Hallucinations	+
	+	Delusions	+
Speech rambling and incoherent		Stereotyped and limited	
Often diurnal variation		Constant (in later stages)	
Often aware and anxious		Unaware and unconcerned (in later stages)	

Be specific!

Patients manifesting the following have all been described as 'confused'

● not taking in what is said:
    deaf
    anxious
    too ill to concentrate

- muddled speech:
    poor concentration
    nominal dysphasia.

It is also important to identify hypnogogic (when going to sleep) and hypnopompic (when waking up) hallucinations as these are normal phenomena, although more common in ill patients receiving sedative drugs.

Causes

Dementia is usually caused by Alzheimer's disease or cerebral atherosclerosis; occasionally it may be paraneoplastic. The causes of other secondary mental disorders are

- drugs
- biochemical derangement
- organ failure
- brain tumours
- paraneoplastic.

Delirium

Delirium (acute confusional state) is the result of mental clouding. This leads to a disturbance of comprehension and bewilderment. Manifestations include

- poor concentration
- impairment of short term memory
- disorientation
- misinterpretations
- paranoid delusions

- hallucinations
- rambling incoherent speech
- restlessness
- noisy/aggressive behaviour.

There may be associated drowsiness. Psychomotor activity may be increased or decreased. Increased activity may be associated with overactivity of the autonomic nervous system, i.e. facial flushing, dilated pupils, injected conjunctivae, tachycardia and sweating.

Delirium is precipitated or exacerbated by many factors (Table 4.19).

Table 4.19: Common precipitating factors for delirium

Change of environment	Constipation
Unfamiliar excessive stimuli	Retention of urine
too hot	Infection
too cold	Dehydration
wet bed	Vitamin deficiency
crumbs in bed	Alcohol deprivation
creases in sheets	Anxiety
Pain and fatigue	Depression

Treatment

The contents of hallucinations, nightmares and misinterpretations tend to reflect the patient's unresolved or recurrent fears and anxieties, and should be explored by skilled questioning.

Explanation

- stress to both the patient and the relatives that the patient is not going mad, and there is a physical cause

- stress that there are usually lucid intervals

- continue to treat the patient with courtesy and respect.

General measures

- restraints should never be used

- bed rails should be avoided – they can be dangerous

- patient should be allowed to walk about accompanied

- allay fear and suspicion, and reduce misinterpretations by:
  use of night light
  not changing the position of the patient's bed
  explaining every procedure and event in detail
  the presence of a family member or close friend.

Drugs

Generally use drugs only if symptoms are marked, persistent and cause distress to the patient and/or family. Review sooner rather than later if a sedative drug is prescribed because symptoms may be exacerbated.

Consider the following measures

- reduction in medication

- oxygen if cyanosed

- dexamethasone if cerebral tumour (see p.147)

- haloperidol 1.5–5 mg PO or SC if agitated, hallucinating or paranoid.

The initial dose of haloperidol depends on previous medication, weight, age and severity of symptoms. Subsequent doses depend on the initial response. Daily or b.d. maintenance doses are usually adequate.

Terminal distress

This is often associated with delirium and may need haloperidol 10–30 mg/24 h and/or midazolam 10–60 mg/24 h by continuous SC infusion to control it.

Occasionally SC phenobarbitone 100–200 mg stat and 800–1600 mg/ 24 h is substituted for haloperidol and midazolam. At some centres, methotrimeprazine is used; this can be regarded as double strength chlorpromazine.

Drug profiles

Corticosteroids

Corticosteroids are used for many reasons in advanced cancer (Table 4.20). Inclusion in the table does *not* mean that a corticosteroid is necessarily the treatment of choice in that situation.

At Sobell House, dexamethasone is the corticosteroid of choice. It is usually given in a single daily dose. Dexamethasone has a duration of effect of 36–54 h, compared with 18–36 h for prednisolone.

Dexamethasone is seven times more potent than prednisolone. Thus, 2 mg of dexamethasone is approximately equivalent to 15 mg of prednisolone. Dexamethasone is available in 0.5 mg and 2 mg tablets, and also as an injection. Prednisolone is available in a range of sizes from 1–25 mg.

The initial daily dose varies according to indication and fashion, ranging from dexamethasone 2–4 mg (prednisolone 15–30 mg) for anorexia to 16–32 mg for spinal cord compression. A dose of 8–16 mg is generally used for raised intracranial pressure.

Oral candidiasis and ankle oedema are common adverse effects. Moonfacing, hyperphagia, weight gain, myopathy or diabetes mellitus

Table 4.20:   Indications for use of corticosteroids in advanced cancer

Specific
Spinal cord compression
Nerve compression
Dyspnoea
   pneumonitis (after radiotherapy)
   carcinomatous lymphangitis
   tracheal compression/stridor
Superior vena caval obstruction
Pericardial effusion
Haemoptysis
Obstruction of hollow viscus
   bronchus
   ureter
   [bowel]
Hypercalcaemia (in corticosteroid responsive tumours, e.g.
lymphoma, myeloma)
Radiation induced inflammation
Leuco-erythroblastic anaemia
Rectal discharge (give PR)
Sweating

Pain relief
Raised intracranial pressure
Nerve compression
Spinal cord compression
Metastatic arthralgia
[Bone pain]

Hormone therapy
Replacement
Anticancer

General
To improve appetite
To enhance sense of wellbeing
To improve strength

may necessitate dose reduction and, sometimes, cessation of treatment.

Agitation, insomnia or a more florid psychiatric disturbance may be precipitated by corticosteroids – either when commencing or stopping treatment.

Apart from hydrocortisone, corticosteroids should normally be given in a single daily dose in the morning to ease compliance and to prevent insomnia. Even so, temazepam or diazepam at bedtime is sometimes needed to counter insomnia or agitation.

Antacids

An antacid is a chemical substance taken by mouth to neutralize gastric acid. Generic antacids include

- sodium bicarbonate
- magnesium salts (cause diarrhoea)
- aluminium hydroxide (causes constipation)
- hydrotalcite (magnesium aluminium carbonate)
- calcium carbonate.

Points to remember

Some antacids contain significant amounts of sodium. This may be important in patients with hypertension or cardiac failure. Liquid Gaviscon (*see overleaf*) and magnesium trisilicate mixture both contain 6.3 mmol/10 ml compared with 0.1 mmol/10 ml in Asilone. Regular use of sodium bicarbonate may cause sodium loading and metabolic alkalosis.

Aluminium hydroxide binds dietary phosphate. It is of benefit in patients with hyperphosphataemia in renal failure. The long term complications of phosphate depletion and osteomalacia are not usually an issue in advanced cancer.

Hydrotalcite binds bile salts and is therefore of specific benefit in patients with bile salt reflux, e.g. after certain forms of gastroduodenal surgery.

Regular use of calcium carbonate may cause hypercalcaemia, particularly if taken with sodium bicarbonate.

Preparations

Proprietary preparations usually contain a mixture of magnesium and aluminium so as to neutralize any effect on the bowels. They may also contain sodium bicarbonate.

Some antacids contain additional substances

- activated dimethicone is an antifoaming agent present in Asilone, a proprietary antacid. By facilitating belching, dimethicone eases flatulence, distension and postprandial gastric distension pain

- alginic acid (Gaviscon) prevents oesophageal reflux pain by forming an inert low density 'raft' on the top of the acid stomach contents. Gaviscon needs both *acid* and *air bubbles* to produce the raft. It may be less effective if used with an H_2 receptor blocker (reduces acid) and/or antiflatulent (reduces air bubbles)

- oxethazaine (in Mucaine) eases reflux pain by coating and anaesthetizing damaged oesophageal mucosa.

Diazepam

Properties and uses

- anxiolytic
- night sedative

- muscle relaxant
- anticonvulsant.

Diazepam is sometimes used as a 'secondary anti-emetic' in patients receiving chemotherapy.

Limitations

- daytime drowsiness
- muscular flaccidity
- postural hypotension.

General comments

- plasma halflife 20–100 h; usually given once a day at *bedtime*. If patient does not sleep at night, daytime drowsiness more likely
- patients occasionally react paradoxically, i.e. become more distressed; if this happens, change to haloperidol or chlorpromazine
- diazepam acts faster PO or PR than IM because the usual preparation is oil-based; IV may cause thrombophlebitis
- if available, use diazepam oil-in-water emulsion (Diazemuls); this is less irritant.

Therapeutic guidelines

Initial dose depends on

- patient's previous experience of diazepam and other benzo-diazepines
- intensity of distress
- urgency of relief.

The following doses are a guide

- 2 mg is useful and safe in the elderly
- 5 mg is the typical initial dose
- 10 mg is useful for severe distress, particularly in younger patients.

Repeat *hourly* until the desired effect is achieved, and then decide on an appropriate maintenance regimen.

Rectal diazepam is useful in a crisis or if the patient is moribund

- suppositories 10 mg
- rectal solution 5–10 mg in 2.5 ml
- parenteral formulation inserted through a cannula.

Patterns of use

- *'as needed'* is the best initial way in the elderly, and for acute (possibly transient) episodes of severe anxiety
- *regularly at bedtime* is best for those with persistent anxiety – to be used as an adjunct to psychological measures. Also if used for muscle spasm or general stiffness
- *more than daily* (e.g. 1000/1400, 2200 h or 1000, 1800, 2200 h) in agitated moribund patients to reduce the number of hours the patient is awake and distressed.

Midazolam

The main advantage of midazolam is that it is water soluble and is miscible with most of the drugs commonly given by continuous SC infusion. It is also easier for IV injection.

Properties and uses

- anaesthetic induction agent
- sedative for minor procedures
- sedative for terminal agitation
- anticonvulsant.

Midazolam versus diazepam

In single doses

- for sedation, midazolam is three times as potent
- as an anticonvulsant, midazolam is twice as potent.

With multiple doses, diazepam will gain in potency because of its prolonged plasma halflife, i.e. 20–100 h versus 1–4 h for midazolam (but about 10 h when given by infusion).

Patterns of use

Typical doses for midazolam are shown in Table 4.21.

Table 4.21: Dose recommendations for SC midazolam

Indication	Stat dose	Initial infusion rate (24 h)	Common range
Muscle relaxant Multifocal myoclonus	5 mg	10 mg	10–30 mg
Terminal agitation Anticonvulsant	10 mg	30 mg	30–60 mg

In terminal agitation, if the patient is not settled on 30 mg/24 h, introduce a neuroleptic drug before increasing the dose of midazolam further.

Haloperidol

Properties and uses

- anti-emetic
- antipsychotic
- anxiolytic.

Limitations

- anticholinergic effects
- extrapyramidal effects
- drowsiness.

General comments

- plasma halflife 12–20 h; can usually be given once daily
- in higher doses (> 5 mg) has a sedative effect, and may substitute satisfactorily for a night sedative
- extrapyramidal effects more likely at daily doses of > 5 mg. Because these do not occur consistently, an antiparkinsonian drug should not be prescribed prophylactically
- anxiolytic of choice if patient hallucinating, paranoid, or in agitated delirium.

Haloperidol versus chlorpromazine

- less sedative
- less anticholinergic effects
- less cardiovascular effects

- more potent anti-emetic
- more extrapyramidal effects.

Therapeutic guidelines

Haloperidol is available in solution, capsule (0.5 mg), tablet (1.5, 5, 10, 20 mg) and parenteral forms.

Anti-emetic (for chemical/toxic causes of vomiting)

- 1.5 mg stat and nocte is standard for vomiting induced by morphine
- 3–5 mg nocte if smaller dose not effective
- 5–30 mg nocte (or in divided dosage) for vomiting induced by chemotherapy and in some patients with hypercalcaemia or uraemia.

Antipsychotic

- 1.5–3 mg stat and nocte in the elderly
- 5 mg stat and nocte in the younger patient or if poor response in the elderly
- 10–30 mg nocte (or in divided dosage) if poor response.

Anxiolytic

- 5 mg stat and nocte
- 10–20 mg nocte (or in divided dosage) if poor response.

Hyoscine

Hyoscine (scopolamine) is an anticholinergic drug with smooth muscle relaxant (antispasmodic) and antisecretory properties. It is available as *hydrobromide* and *butylbromide* (Buscopan) salts. The latter is a quaternary salt and does not cross the blood-brain barrier. Unlike hyoscine *hydrobromide*, hyoscine *butylbromide* does not cause somnolence, nor does it have a central anti-emetic action.

- hyoscine *butylbromide* is poorly absorbed PO. By this route it is of use only in bowel colic
- repeated administration of hyoscine *hydrobromide* leads to cumulation and may result paradoxically in an agitated delirium. If this occurs, add diazepam or midazolam.

Preparations

Hyoscine hydrobromide

- SL 0.3 mg (Quick Kwell)
- SC 0.4 mg, 0.6 mg
- transdermal patch 0.5 mg over 3 days.

Hyoscine butylbromide

- PO 10 mg
- SC 20 mg.

Therapeutic guidelines

Injections of hyoscine *butylbromide* are cheaper than hyoscine *hydrobromide* and should generally be used in preference. The main indications are

- 'death rattle'
- bowel obstruction (*see* p.115).

Hyoscine *hydrobromide* by any route and hyoscine *butylbromide* SC can also be used in other situations where an anticholinergic drug may be beneficial, e.g. sialorrhoea.

Despite a plasma halflife of about 8 h, the duration of antisecretory effect is only about 1 h (*butylbromide*) and 2 h (*hydrobromide*). Thus, for this purpose, best given as a transdermal patch or by continuous SC infusion.

Anticholinergic (antimuscarinic) effects

'dry as a bone,
blind as a bat,
red as a beet,
hot as a hare,
mad as a hatter'

Several drugs used in palliative care have anticholinergic properties (Table 4.22).

Table 4.22:   Anticholinergic drugs

Belladonna alkaloids
  atropine
  hyoscine
	Antihistamines
	  chlorpheniramine
	  cyclizine
	  dimenhydrinate
	  promethazine

Glycopyrronium	

Neuroleptics
  butyrophenones
  (haloperidol, droperidol)
  phenothiazines
	Antispasmodics
	  mebeverine
	  oxybutynin
	  propantheline

Tricyclic antidepressants	

Anticholinergic effects may be a limiting factor in symptom management. The concurrent use of two anticholinergic drugs should be avoided, if possible. A list of anticholinergic effects is given in Table 4.23.

Table 4.23: Anticholinergic effects

Visual

Mydriasis
Loss of accommodation } blurred vision

Cardiovascular

Palpitations
Extrasystoles } also related to noradrenaline potentiation
Arrhythmias } and a quinidine-like action

Gastro-intestinal

Dry mouth
Heartburn (reduced tone in lower oesophageal sphincter)
Constipation

Urinary tract

Hesitancy of micturition
Retention of urine

When all's said and done
Professional carers have needs too

When all's said and done

Caring for the dying is full of paradoxes. One general practitioner wrote, 'I have looked after several patients who have died at home. I still find it extremely harrowing but very rewarding.'

Another doctor said to a patient's wife as he left the house, 'I don't know why I keep visiting, I never do anything.' To which the wife replied, 'Oh, Doctor Smith, don't say that! If only you knew the difference your visits make to us'.

Palliative care developed as a reaction to the attitude, spoken or unspoken, that 'there is nothing more that we can do for you' with the inevitable consequence for the patient and family of a sense of abandonment, hopelessness and despair. It was stressed that this was never true – there is always something that can be done. Even so, there are times when the doctor or nurse *feels* that he/she has nothing to offer. In this circumstance one is thrown back on who one is as an individual. Sheila Cassidy has illustrated this in a series of sketches (Figures 5.1–5.4).

'Slowly, I learn about the importance of powerlessness.
I experience it in my own life and I live with it in my work.
The secret is not to be afraid of it – not to run away.
The dying know we are not God.
All they ask is that we do not desert them.'[33]

Figure 5.1: This shows the doctor, armed with his competence and his instruments and protected by his aide.[33] (Figures 5.1 to 5.4 are reproduced with permission from Cassidy S (1988) *Sharing the darkness*. Darton, Longman and Todd.)

Figure 5.2: A priest performing his sacramental ministry. Here we see him wearing his stole and clerical collar protected by having a role to play and a ritual to perform.[33]

Figure 5.3:   A patient meeting with either doctor or clergyman when he has exhausted the physical aspects of his ministry. He is left with his hands empty – but with his resources of counselling still available.[33]

Figure 5.4:   Both patient and carer stripped of their resources, present to each other, naked and empty handed, as two human beings.[33]

When there is nothing to offer except ourselves, a belief that life has meaning and purpose helps to sustain the carer. However, to speak glibly of this to a patient who is in despair is cruel. At such times, actions speak louder than words. By what is done, the essential message is conveyed:

> 'You matter because you are you. You matter to the last moment of your life, and we will do all we can not only to help you die peacefully, but to live until you die.'[34]

As someone observed:

> 'Those who have the strength and the love to sit with a dying patient in the silence that goes beyond words will know that this moment is neither frightening nor painful, but a peaceful cessation of the functioning of the body.
>
> Watching a peaceful death of a human being reminds us of a falling star, one of the millions of lights in a vast sky that flares up for a brief moment only to disappear into the endless night forever.'[35]

Professional carers have needs too

Palliative care places many stresses on the professional carer. These include

- coping with the failure of medical cure
- repeated exposure to the death of people with whom we have formed a relationship
- involvement in emotional conflicts
- absorption of anger being expressed

- role-blurring in multiprofessional teamwork

- personal idealism

- challenges to personal belief systems.

The following are prerequisites for self-care[36]

- love

- self-esteem

- a body image you accept

- a wish to develop creativity

- imagination

- flexibility

- humour

- compassion

- a capacity to accept mistakes and the ability to correct them

- a mind ready to take challenges.

> 'Caring is an ongoing creative process. If creativity is arrested or stopped, caring and hope are not possible. You have to restore creativity in order to restore hope.'[36]

A range of strategies helps to preserve emotional and physical health and avoid 'burnout'

- work as a team:
  shared decisions and responsibility
  mutual support and respect

- good communication within the team

- good resources and support services

- realistic goals

- be open to receive support from your patients
- adequate off-duty/food/rest
- time for recreation:
    hobbies
    spiritual refreshment.

Sometimes it is helpful to have the support of an outside professional counsellor, clinical psychologist or psychotherapist. There are many opportunities for personal growth within the challenges of palliative care. These challenges can be welcomed despite often being painful

- facing one's own mortality
- facing one's own limitations personally and professionally
- sharing control
- learning to be with patients, not just doing things for them
- facing challenges to one's own beliefs
- dealing honestly with personal emotions, e.g. anger, grief, hurt.

References

1 Wood CB (1984) In: CJH Van den Velde and PH Sugarbaker (eds) *Liver metastases*. Martinus Nijhoff, Dordrecht. pp 47–54.

2 Pettingale KW *et al.* (1985) Mental attitudes to cancer: an additional prognostic factor. *Lancet.* **i**: 750.

3 Frank A (1991) *At the will of the body: reflections on illness.* Houghton Mifflin, Boston.

4 Calman KC (1984) Quality of life in cancer patients – an hypothesis. *Journal of Medical Ethics.* **10**: 124–127.

5 Van Dam FSAM *et al.* (1984) Evaluating 'quality of life' in cancer clinical trials. In: ME Buyse *et al.* (eds) *Cancer clinical trials: methods and practice.* Oxford University Press, Oxford. pp 26–43.

6 Twycross RG (1987) Quality before quantity – a note of caution. *Palliative Medicine.* **1**: 65–72.

7 Cohen SR and Mount BM (1992) Quality of life in terminal illness: defining and measuring subjective well-being in the dying. *Journal of Palliative Care.* **8** (3): 40–45.

8 Gillon R (1994) Medical ethics: four principles plus attention to scope. *British Medical Journal.* **309**: 84–188.

9 Lunt B and Neale C (1987) A comparison of hospice and hospital: care goals set by staff. *Palliative Medicine.* **1**: 136–148.

10 Herth K (1990) Fostering hope in terminally-ill people. *Journal of Advanced Nursing.* **15**: 1250–1259.

11 Simpson MA (1979) *The facts of death.* Prentice-Hall, Englewood Cliffs, New Jersey.

12 Parkes CM (1972) Accuracy of predictions of survival in later stages of cancer. *British Medical Journal.* **ii**: 29–33.

13 Spiritual Care Working Group (1994) Sir Michael Sobell House, Oxford.

14 Kubotera T (1988) Personal communication.

15 Speck P (1984) *Being there: pastoral care in time of illness.* SPCK, London.

16 Department of Health (1991) *The patient's charter.* HMSO, London.

17 Gatrad AR (1994) Muslim customs surrounding death, bereavement, postmortem examinations, and organ transplants. *British Medical Journal.* **309**: 521–523.

18 Green J (1989) Hinduism. *Nursing Times.* **85** (6): 50–51.

19 Green J (1989) Buddhism. *Nursing Times.* **85** (9): 40–41.

20 Allingham M (1957) *The tiger in the smoke.* Penguin, Harmondsworth.

21 Campbell AB Quoted in: O'Toole D (1987) *Healing and growing through grief.* Blue Cross and Blue Shield, Michigan.

22 O'Toole D (1987) *Healing and growing through grief.* Blue Cross and Blue Shield, Michigan.

23 Parkes CM (1986) *Bereavement: studies of grief in adult life.* (2nd edn) Pelican, London.

24 Worden JW (1991) *Grief counselling and grief therapy.* (2nd edn) Tavistock, London.

25 Le Poidevin S Unpublished material.

26 Parkes CM (1990) Risk factors in bereavement: implications for the prevention and treatment of pathologic grief. *Psychiatric Annals.* **20**: 308–313.

27 Osterweiss M, Solomon F and Morris G (eds) (1984) *Bereavement reactions: consequences and care.* National Academy Press, Washington.

28 Raphael B (1977) Preventive intervention with the recently bereaved. *Archives of General Psychiatry.* **34**: 1450–1454.

29 Yaniv H (1994) Personal communication.

30 International Association for the Study of Pain Task Force on Taxonomy (1994) *Classification of chronic pain.* (2nd edn) IASP Press, Seattle.

31 World Health Organization (1986) *Cancer pain relief.* WHO, Geneva.

32 Krebs HB and Goplerud DR (1987) Mechanical intestinal obstruction in patients with gynecologic disease: A review of 368 patients. *American Journal of Obstetrics and Gynecology.* **157**: 577–583.

33 Cassidy S (1988) *Sharing the darkness.* Darton, Longman and Todd, London. pp 61–64.

34 Saunders C Unpublished talk.

35 Kubler-Ross E (1969) *On death and dying.* Tavistock, London.

36 Bild R (1994) Personal communication.

Further reading
Specific

Doyle D, Hanks GW and MacDonald N (eds) (1994) *Oxford textbook of palliative medicine.* Oxford University Press, Oxford.

Stedeford A (1994) *Facing death: patients, families and professionals.* (2nd edn) Sobell Publications, Oxford.

Twycross RG (1994) *Pain relief in advanced cancer.* Churchill Livingstone, Edinburgh.

Twycross RG and Lack SA (1993) *Oral morphine in advanced cancer.* (Revised 2nd edn) Beaconsfield Publishers, Beaconsfield.

General

Barraclough J (1994) *Cancer and emotion.* John Wiley, Chichester.

Cassidy S (1988) *Sharing the darkness.* Darton, Longman and Todd, London.

Frank A (1991) *At the will of the body: reflections on illness.* Houghton Mifflin, Boston.

Frankl V (1959) *Man's search for meaning.* Simon and Shuster, New York.

Hill S (1974) *In the springtime of the year.* Penguin Books, London.

Lewis CS (1961) *A grief observed.* Faber and Faber, London.

Peck SM (1990) *The road less travelled: a new psychology of love, traditional values and spiritual growth.* Arrow Books, London.

Working Party Report (1991) *Mud and stars. The impact of hospice experience on the church's ministry of healing.* Sobell Publications, Oxford.

Index